# The Hormone Healing Cookbook

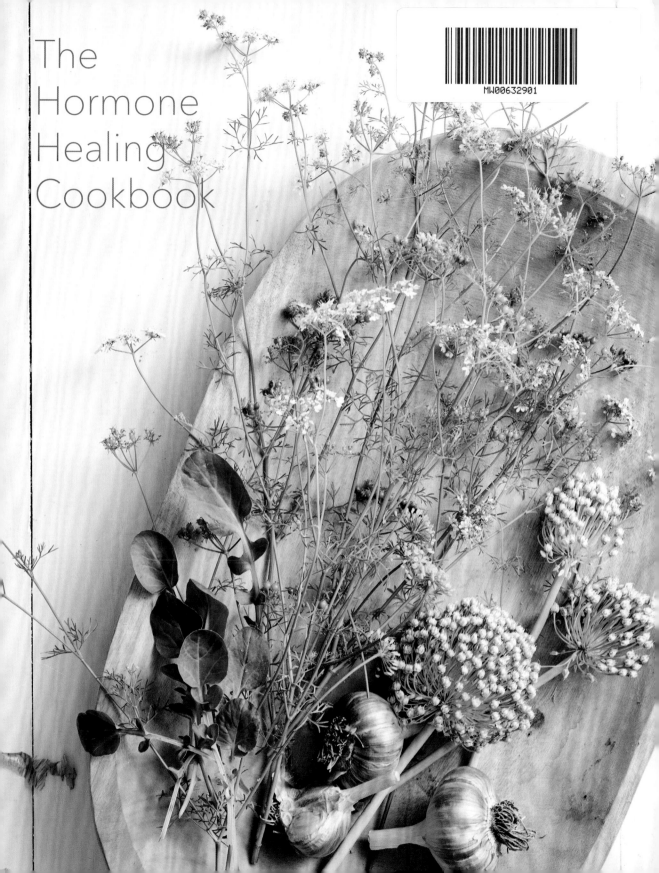

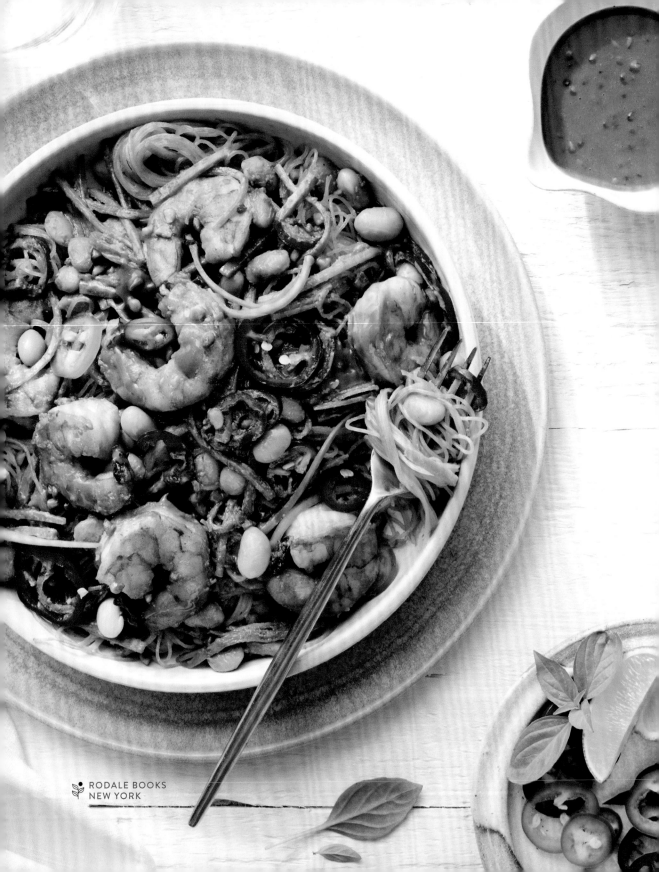

RODALE BOOKS
NEW YORK

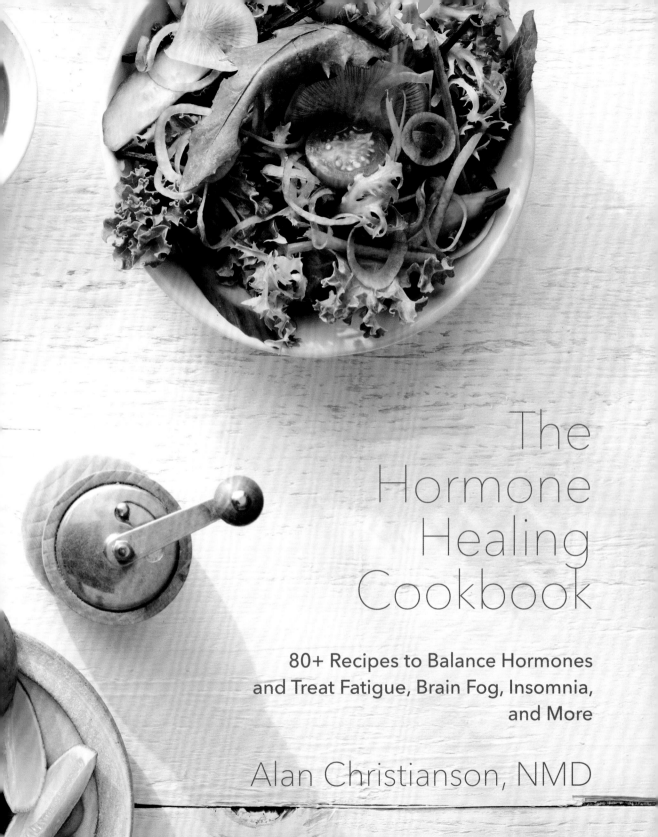

# The Hormone Healing Cookbook

## 80+ Recipes to Balance Hormones and Treat Fatigue, Brain Fog, Insomnia, and More

Alan Christianson, NMD

Published in the United States by Rodale Books, an imprint of Random House, a division of Penguin Random House LLC, New York.
RodaleBooks.com
RandomHouseBooks.com

RODALE and the Plant colophon are registered trademarks of Penguin Random House LLC.

Library of Congress Cataloging-in-Publication Data

Names: Christianson, Alan, author. Title: The hormone healing cookbook : 80+ recipes to balance hormones and treat fatigue, brain fog, insomnia, and more / by Alan Christianson, NMD. Description: First edition. | New York : Rodale, [2023] | Includes bibliographical references. | Identifiers: LCCN 2022030666 | ISBN 9780593235812 (trade paperback) | ISBN 9780593235829 (ebook). Subjects: LCSH: Weight loss—Endocrine aspects—Popular works. | Endocrine glands—Diseases—Diet therapy—Popular works. | Metabolism—Regulation—Popular works.
Classification: LCC RM222.2 .C48394 2023 | DDC 641.5/63—dc23/eng /20220802
LC record available at https://lccn .loc.gov/2022030666

ISBN 978-0-593-23581-2
Ebook ISBN 978-0-593-23582-9

Printed in China

Photographer: Jennifer Chong
Photography Assistant: David Peng
Food Stylist: Laura Kinsey Dolph
Assistant Food Stylist: Courtney Weis
Prop Stylist: Alicia Buszczak
Editor: Michele Eniclerico
Assistant Editor: Danielle Curtis

Designers: Zaiah Sampson, Jen Wang
Cover Designer: Zaiah Sampson
Cover Photographs: Jennifer Chong
Production Editor: Patricia Shaw
Production Manager: Kelli Tokos
Compositor: Merri Ann Morrell and dix!
Copy Editor: Nancy Inglis
Marketer: Jamila Coleman
Publicist: Lindsey Kennedy

10 9 8 7 6 5 4 3 2 1

First Edition

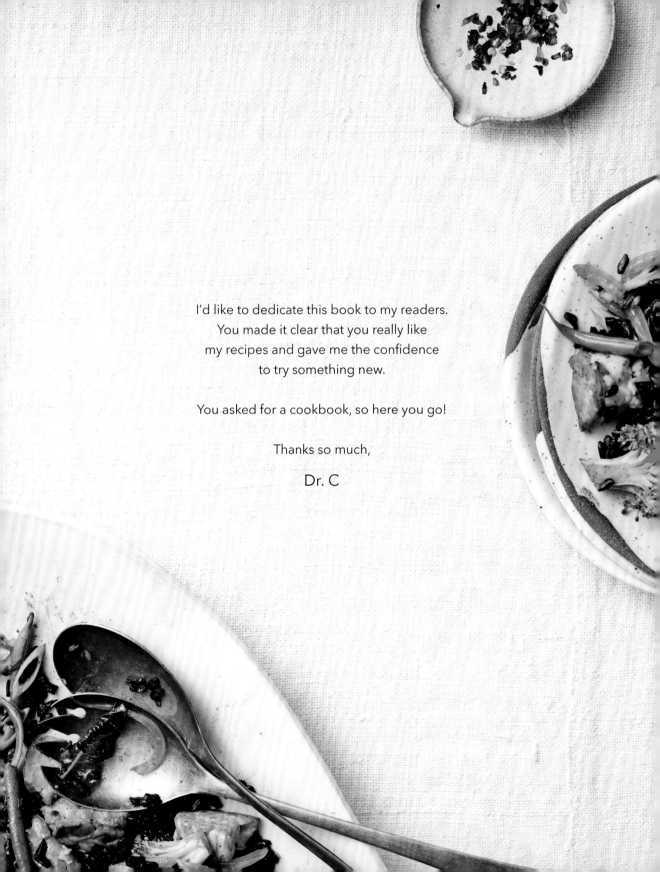

I'd like to dedicate this book to my readers.
You made it clear that you really like
my recipes and gave me the confidence
to try something new.

You asked for a cookbook, so here you go!

Thanks so much,

Dr. C

# Contents

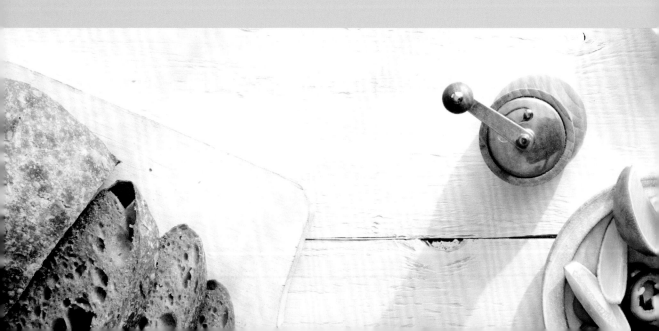

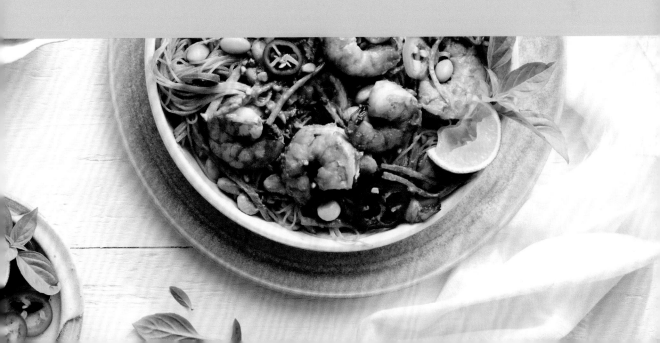

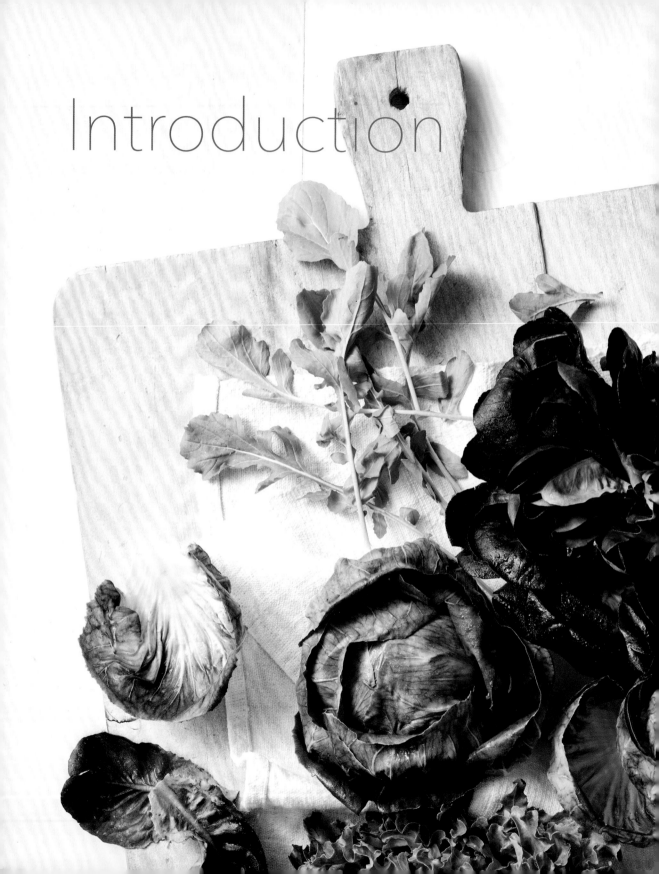

Introduction

# Why a Cookbook?

I believe that good health is an essential ingredient in a good life. I believe that the key to one's best health is a lifestyle based on deliberate habits supported by solid evidence. That includes a diet with a variety of minimally processed foods in reasonable amounts. But that's not the end of the story. You can tailor that diet to further meet your specific needs, and I'm honored to show you how in *The Hormone Healing Cookbook*.

My first book to reach a wider audience contained the idea that foods could be timed in a way to reset the body's stress response. It included meal plans and recipes to provide practical applications. I was excited to share the idea. It seemed to me to be a big idea, a revolutionary one. I've always enjoyed healthful cooking, and it seemed like an afterthought to plug in some of my favorite recipes.

My readers' feedback surprised me. They did find the program to be helpful, and they shared inspiring results. I was elated but also pleasantly surprised to learn that the recipes were a big part of their success.

I started sharing more recipes online, along with publishing two more books. Still, readers asked for a cookbook.

Well, I've finally delivered! And while there's no way to deny that this book is all about the easy, delicious recipes, they are all in service to one idea: that specific foods can reverse a hormone imbalance and your symptoms can illuminate which foods to focus on. Daily cooking is more than a way to feed yourself. It is the center of a healthy and happy life.

The better your life is, the fewer preventable issues emerge, and the better you can deal with the unpreventable ones.

From our surveys and from the questions you've sent, your top concerns are weight loss, more energy, better mental function, easier menopause, and improved sleep. Some of these have been covered in my other books; others have not. The common thread is that these are all hormonal symptoms.

Let me expand on the word *hormone* so we can be sure we're talking about the same thing.

In the medical world, hormones are chemicals that regulate the body's systems. The most relevant ones include hormones from the thyroid, the adrenal glands, and the ovaries or testicles. When people outside medical circles talk about hormones, they usually mean estrogen-related symptoms like PMS, menopause, or fertility. When this cookbook talks about hormones, it means all of the above. There is so much research showing that food can help hormone regulation, and I'm excited to share it with you in a practical form.

There are three ways to make use of these recipes. First, this cookbook is organized around top hormonal symptoms. If you're struggling mainly with one of these symptoms—weight gain, fatigue, brain fog, insomnia, or hot flashes—follow one of the 14-Day Menu Plans to get relief (starting on page 70). Second, you can use these as recipes for the programs in other books. Some need a little modification, which I have provided. Third is to just skip around and have fun. Find a recipe that sounds good, give it a try, and repeat. They are all tasty, easy, and healthy.

## Why Symptoms?

I organized this cookbook around symptoms because they are what matter most.

All too often the medical world focuses on everything but symptoms, when the whole point is to help you feel better. Doctors often focus on laboratory results over symptoms because symptoms are out of their control. They can't assign numbers to them, and symptoms can get worse even if doctors prescribe the "right" treatment.

Lab findings are part of the doctors' sphere of control. Symptoms are not. When patients talk about symptoms, they are the ones in control. When the focus is on labs, the doctor can decide whether the treatment worked or not. Did the lab results get better? Then case closed.

But there is no victory unless your symptoms improve. You don't really care if your labs are better if you don't *feel* better. Symptoms are more than different forms of discomfort. They can determine the quality of your life. They are also the best way for you to know what is happening inside your body. If they persist, you know there is still an underlying problem that has been missed.

The fewer of them you have and the milder they are, the better your life is. As an endocrinologist, I focus on the hormones behind the symptoms. Is the culprit estrogen, cortisol, or T3 from the thyroid? There is a

place for this approach, but it has its limits. The typical scenario is that doctors will rule out the most severe diseases and then proclaim that nothing else is wrong. They are often not trained to think about hormones. Symptoms are the first sign of a hormone imbalance. Disease is the second sign.

The body adjusts its hormone levels to stay in balance. Hormones govern the rate and the timing of our core chemical reactions. When reactions occur too slowly, we feel tired, gain weight, and can't think clearly. When the timing of daily reactions is disrupted, we can't sleep well. Timing also applies to how well we move through life's stages like perimenopause and menopause. If the events within these major transitions are not smoothly orchestrated, normal symptoms of the transition are worse.

There is a balancing act between doing what you can to improve your own health and seeking medical care when appropriate. The only simple answer to this dilemma is to have a good working relationship with a health care professional. Even when you have a good relationship, there are times when you need to decide whether to focus on self-care or further diagnosis. Consider a second opinion if your symptoms are severe, new, or changing, or if you feel your symptoms aren't being taken seriously. If your symptoms are stable and well explained, but you're still not feeling your best, you can now take matters into your own kitchen. Cooking is powerful. I say this because I've seen food help tens of thousands of people over the course of more than twenty-five years of patient care. This cookbook draws on my experience and the medical literature to select specific foods to help these top hormonal symptoms.

But food is just the starting place. For the recipes to work, they must become part of your daily life. If food is to be an effective solution, it must be easy to find and work with. Most of all, the meals must taste good. Some people might be able to force themselves to eat things they don't like or skip their favorite foods for longer than others, but no one can do it long term. The right food can help, but only if it is part of a good recipe and a lifestyle that works for you. It can help even more when the recipe is tailored to your specific symptoms. Every recipe in this cookbook was created to help you feel better. The ingredients were chosen because of their specific effects. And, if you'll forgive me for saying so myself, they are good!

I think we can agree that good food is fresh, flavorful, balanced, properly cooked, and lovingly prepared. Good food is satisfying, nourishing, and good for you. It leaves you feeling alive and eager to take on life's challenges. If you don't already love to cook, this cookbook might change that. Making meal plans and shopping lists can be the hardest part, and I've done that for you! When it involves less struggle, cooking can be a form of meditation.

Cooking can be a daily reset, a time to become aware and deliberate, and it requires heightened awareness. It demands you to be in touch with all your senses. What is the right color for onions that have been properly sweated? How should a sizzle sound when the pan is hot enough? What does *done* smell like?

If you make cooking a habit, you will drop into a meditative state once you launch into it. It will force you to break away from nagging thoughts and worries. You'll connect more deeply with those you're cooking for. Soon you'll choose foods based on how you know they will make you feel rather than out of habit or boredom.

I started to think about how important food was when I was twelve. My birth mother had too much going against her to keep me. Some of her issues likely contributed to mine. I was born with frequent seizures and problems with coordination. I could not do things like play sports, draw, or write legibly. As we all do, I automatically played to my strengths. Books were mine. I read at an early age, and my greatest pleasure was the excitement of wrapping my head around something new. I was happy with my books and ideas.

But everything changed during my adolescence. I got heavier, and peers became more important. They rejected me because of my weight, and I in turn rejected myself. I felt disgusting and unacceptable. I was still into books, and they saved me again. I knew exactly where all the books about space were in the local library. One time as I was heading toward that section, a book's title caught my eye. It was called *Let's Get Healthy*. That book changed the arc of my life. Even just seeing the title shifted my mindset. It implied that you could *choose* your health. That idea was new to me. Up until that point, my poor health seemed like something that just happened to me, like the weather.

I took the book off the shelf and read nearly all of it while standing right there. I implemented what I could. After all, I was still a kid, so there was only so much I could do. I didn't have any supplements. Food was what Mom cooked and what she stocked in our pantry. In retrospect, I have to say we did not have a lot of junk food and my mom made good meals. I was filling up too much on snacks and not enough on protein, veggies, and good carbs. I did not cook yet, but I had some leeway in my choices. Mom had protein powder in the pantry, so I started having it for breakfast. I chose what and how much I put on my plate for dinner. I had the power to decline sweets and extra servings.

These small choices helped, teaching me critical lessons. I learned that happiness requires health, and health requires good food. From them, I started to develop confidence that allowed me to start exercising. I discovered that my prior physical limits were no longer as relevant. What was holding me back was my sedentary habits. I changed this behavior and I flourished.

As I grew older, my latitude over food choices increased. Mom let me help and taught me how to cook. Soon I started to help with cooking and shopping. One of my favorite memories was a weekend I spent with my grandma Christianson. She wanted to pass on to me some of my family's favorite recipes, like lefse (a large thin potato pancake) and meatballs. In fact, a lot of the recipes here drew on my mom's "cookbook," a shoebox filled with heirloom recipes from lovely Scandinavian women. They are all handwritten and on various sizes of paper. I know they have seen actual use because many are stained from lying out on a busy kitchen counter.

By the time I was sixteen, I had started working as a cook. It was a great high school job, but I wanted to use food and other natural methods to help people feel better. This path led me to become a naturopathic physician and eventually a naturopathic endocrinologist.

Sadly, I did not cook much during my first few years of practice. I was working seventy plus hours a week to get things going. Because I managed my schedule so poorly, all my food ended up coming from packages or restaurants. Even though I made "good" choices, I wasn't getting good food. Exercise was also put on the back burner. I went from being a daily exerciser to being an occasional weekend warrior. Nothing bad happened overnight, but it happened. I was helping people get healthy, while my own health was going the wrong way. My weight went up and my attitude went down. What should have been a happy time was often a struggle.

One day I saw a picture my wife took of me at a family reunion. It was a profile from the side, and I looked like I'd swallowed a basketball! I was totally shocked, but once the problem was clear, I knew I had to start doing the same things I told everybody else to do. Back to daily cooking and exercise. But life was busy, and I had to learn to do it more efficiently. It had to work with time for my family and my career. It was not simple, but it was necessary, and I made it happen.

Of course, these changes took time. But I started feeling better in the first few days. My mood bounced right back up and life was good again. After I got back on track, I was so happy with the results I wanted to share them with my patients. But most of the time I spent with them in the clinic was focused on their medical issues. There was no time to talk about recipes. So I started a blog. This was in the late nineties and the internet was in its infancy.

Ever since, I've loved sharing recipes and learning from others. Over the years I've been lucky enough to cook alongside many other passionate cooks and professional chefs. I've had stages where I've gotten into exotic cuisines, unusual ingredients, and cutting-edge cooking methods. I'll share a couple of these things for fun, but daily cooking should be simple and familiar.

How can this work for you? Think about the top symptoms, pick which you would like to focus on first, and commit to the corresponding meal plan for two weeks. Be receptive to trying a few new ingredients. None are hard to find, but some may be foods you don't eat often.

How hard will it be? Here is what you can expect. Allow fifteen to thirty minutes each day to cook. Each week expect an hour to shop and an hour to prep foods. You can also do the bulk of the work on the weekend. I love to be in the kitchen on Sunday afternoons prepping food and precooking what I can. It is amazing how much more efficient it is to make several things in one session.

Consider journaling during the process as well. Make a note of your discoveries. Which recipes do you really love? How attentive are you in the kitchen? How will you do a recipe differently? What ingredients might you replace to better fit your preferences?

In the first couple of chapters, I'll explain more of the story behind symptoms, hormones, and food. In the next five chapters, we'll talk in depth about these five symptoms—what they mean, what else can contribute to them, which foods help the most, and how over-the-counter supplements can be useful.

In the last two chapters, the bulk of the book, you'll find meal plans, shopping lists, and recipes! As you look through things, the most important point I'd like you to remember is that you *can* heal.

If you have forgotten what it is like to feel good, change can be hard at first. It is too easy to think that you're stuck and can't do anything about it. It takes a leap of faith to get started. If that seems hard, all I ask for is two weeks. Your new routine won't take discipline—it will become automatic. As valuable as health is, you may also find there is more to the journey. Taking these steps can give you self-control and confidence that help in countless ways. All that can start with a few recipes.

In the first chapter, I'll explain how hormonal balance, food, and symptoms are all part of the same package. Let's dive in!

# PART 1

# HORMONES, SYMPTOMS & FOOD

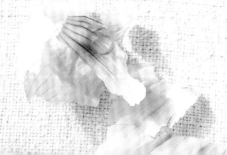

# Hormones & Symptoms

Many people have troublesome symptoms that make them wonder if their hormones are off. Maybe their weight gain doesn't make sense, or they can't figure out why they are so tired. Maybe it is the hot flashes that seem so much worse than what their mom had.

Hormones regulate our chemistry in ways that keep the body healthy. When they're out of balance, they contribute to common and troublesome symptoms like weight gain, fatigue, hot flashes, insomnia, and brain fog.

There are many different types of hormone imbalances that can cause these top five symptoms. Weight gain can point to problems in the thyroid or the adrenals. Fatigue can be abnormal dehydroepiandrosterone (or DHEA, a hormone your body naturally produces in the adrenal glands) or low testosterone. Hot flashes can come from rapid changes in estradiol and progesterone. Insomnia is often the result of melatonin and cortisol not getting along. Brain fog can come from the liver ignoring glucagon from the pancreas.

To help you rebalance your hormones, *The Hormone Healing Cookbook* relies on plant foods that are rich in phytonutrients. Even though we do not develop a deficiency or diseases without them, our bodies rely on phytonutrients for homeostasis. Hormone imbalances arise from an inability to self-regulate. Hormones require many systems of internal regulation, and most of these systems work only in the presence of phytonutrients. A diet rich in the right phytonutrients improves hormone levels because it helps the body to make its own adjustments. People don't get enough phytonutrients in the standard American diet or on a highly restrictive "healthy" diet.

Modern American foods are highly processed. Much of the processing is done to make food tastier and to ensure that it has a longer shelf life. The main examples are white flour, table sugar, and refined oils. We all know these foods are too tasty for our own good, as well as high in calories and low in vitamins. They are also devoid of phytonutrients. Scientists are questioning whether these foods are innately harmful or if they cause harm because they displace foods higher in phytonutrients.

These problems can occur to some people even on "healthy" diets. Many popular diets are highly restrictive. Along with cutting out junk food, some regimens take it too far and cut out some of the healthiest plant foods. So why would the stuff in plants help our hormones?

The reason is that plants make hormones themselves, even some of the same ones that we do. Because of that, the chemicals they make to regulate their hormones also regulate ours when we eat them. Melatonin is one example we'll talk about in chapter 7, "Insomnia." Humans and plants both have a circadian rhythm, and they both make melatonin to regulate it. When we eat melatonin from plants, it affects our circadian rhythm. Estrogens are another example. Humans and plants both use estrogen-like compounds to control growth and reproduction. Estrogens from plants are called phytoestrogens. When we ingest them, they can reduce symptoms from changes in estrogen during menopause.

It seems that the systems that regulate human hormones evolved with the presence of phytonutrients. Our bodies came to depend on these plant compounds. To consume less of them is harmful, but in ways that are not immediately obvious. Modern life is fraught with factors that lead to hormone imbalances. Remember that hormones regulate our bodies. They control our energy production, daily schedules, and reparative processes. Modern life makes all those systems harder to regulate.

In today's world, our schedules are often erratic. We no longer wake and sleep to the sun's rhythm. Our energy production gets thrown off from stimulants, processed foods, snacking, and irregular mealtimes. Tissue repair is harder due to prolonged bouts of inactivity. Of course, stress goes along with all these issues, and it makes everything worse.

Our bodies have many ways of regulating hormones even without phytonutrients. If life ran along more smoothly, our own built-in systems might do okay. But all too often, it does not. The anxieties of modern life put too much stress on our bodies, so our hormones can't stay in balance without the additional help from phytonutrients. Over long periods of time, a lack of hormone regulation leads to our top symptoms, and it also leads to a higher risk of chronic diseases. Food helps hormonal symptoms because it fixes the underlying problems. It's not just a Band-Aid approach that makes things feel better for a while.

There are certainly other diets that purport to balance hormones. How is the approach in *The Hormone Healing Cookbook* different? you might ask. What differentiates this approach is the assumptions those other diets are built on. Are people healthier because of what they add to their diets or what they subtract from them?

It depends on where they start. If someone is on a diet that has too much food in general, and highly processed food at that, they will likely feel better cutting some of it out. But if they do, was it because they cut out bad food or because they replaced it with good food? Some believe so strongly in the benefit of subtraction, they keep on going after the junk food has gone. Some popular approaches avoid entire food groups of natural foods and even large numbers of fruits and vegetables. One popular diet even avoids most plant foods.

These diets assume that many natural foods are bad because they have harmful chemicals. They argue that health comes largely from avoiding bad foods, and they consider many natural, unprocessed foods to be "bad." Some of the items they encourage avoiding include foods high in oxalates, like spinach, almonds, and dates; foods with lectins, such as walnuts, lentils, and brown rice; and nightshade family foods, such as garlic, tomatoes, and eggplant.

Much of the inspiration from these guidelines come from the fact that all these compounds are harmful. Yet the dose makes the poison. In all cases, the harm happens only when you ingest them in concentrations not found in normal foods.

For example, lectins from dried beans can be harmful if the beans are not cooked. Like many nightshades, eggplant contains alkaloids like nicotine, but only about a hundred thousandth as much as cigarettes. Oxalates can build up in our tissues, but our bodies already make more than we could ever absorb from our diets.

I'm not saying these diets are unhelpful in every case. In fact, many people can even go on these diets and find them beneficial. How is this possible? It depends on where they start. If a person is on a standard American diet, or SAD (low in fiber, fruits, and veggies, and high in fat and sugar), they may go on a restrictive diet and feel better at first. They may end up eating fewer processed foods, more vegetables, and more fiber.

It is easy to rely on chemical theories, test tube studies, or animal studies and prove almost anything. The world of biochemistry is so vast, it is possible to have any number of seemingly plausible theories that turn out not to be true. Yet when we look at human studies, things become clearer. If you compare the health of large groups of people who eat a wider range of health foods, they do better than those who have a more restrictive diet. Foods rich in phytonutrients confer better health. This holds true even when we include lectins, oxalates, and nightshade foods. We now know that some things that are dangerous in high doses are actually beneficial in smaller amounts. It turns out that these "dangerous" chemicals in natural foods may be more than harmless. They may be part of what makes the foods healthy.

True, natural foods contain thousands of chemicals, many of which can be dangerous if consumed in large amounts. But the amounts found in food are tiny. By no coincidence, these amounts are exactly enough to keep us healthy. Food is powerful because we co-evolved with it. We domesticated the plants that tasted good and filled us up. We chose the best from each harvest and used their seeds for the next. We gave them protection from insects and weeds, and they kept us healthy. We evolved together.

Broccoli is a great example. We see it as a mundane food, yet it did not exist in the recent past. Some 3,000 years ago, people started cultivating wild cabbage. It was barely edible and had little nutritional value—mostly just tough and bitter leaves. Each crop had a few plants that had larger flower stalks that were not as bitter. That was the one used for the next crop, which would be just a little better. The best example of it was used for the following season. Over thousands of years, wild cabbage became the modern vegetable we refer to as broccoli.

There's a good reason that we don't like foods that are too bitter—they might be poisonous. Plants are loaded with a variety of different poisons, and not by accident. These poisons prevent other plants from growing too close, keep insects from eating the plants they are found in, and give animals diarrhea so they spread their seeds more effectively.

Wild cabbage and broccoli both include poisons called glucosinolates. These compounds are used today as effective pesticides against moths and beetles.[1] As humans selected for better-tasting plants, the amount of glucosinolate in the plant decreased,

but some remains. About 25 percent of the population has genes that make them more sensitive to the taste of some glucosinolates. These people are called supertasters and are more likely to avoid cruciferous vegetables. Glucosinolates in broccoli cause our liver to work harder. They stimulate liver pathways that break them down so that we will be better prepared next time. Those same pathways are used to adjust our hormones. Because humans ingested glucosinolates for so long, our livers don't work well without them.

Evidence suggests that broccoli lowers cancer risks.[2] It is probably more accurate to say that a *lack* of broccoli raises the risks. There are similar stories for many other categories of foods: grains, legumes, nuts, seeds, fruits, and other vegetables. Now you see why the healthiest people are those who eat a full variety of these foods.

*The Hormone Healing Cookbook* treats food as an ally, not as an enemy. It does not attempt to exclude phytonutrients. It uses them to boost the body back to a state of hormonal balance. If it feels like something is not right with your hormones, please know that you can do something about it. You can make daily decisions that bring you the health you want. I wrote this cookbook to help you with one of these decisions: What should you cook tonight?

Too often food has become just another point of controversy. The idea of simple, healthy food can get lost under the noise of the extreme fads. Should you go paleo or vegan? Should you have a breakfast of champions or time-restricted feeding? Is spinach a superfood or a bearer of inflammatory oxalates? The arguments about the health benefits of food are real. The arguments about the hidden dangers of natural foods are not.

The benefit we know the most about is hormone regulation. We need phytonutrients to maintain hormone balance. This cookbook uses phytonutrient-rich recipes to help with the top five symptoms of a hormone imbalance: stubborn weight, fatigue, brain fog, hot flashes, and poor sleep.

It uses solid evidence to help you choose food based on your physical symptoms. Would you like more energy to complete a project? Start the day with a recipe for fatigue like the Beet Green Smoothie on page 109. Are hot flashes making it hard to sleep? For dinner, try the Creamy Shrimp and Tofu Soup on page 142. Has weight been a struggle? Try the 14-Day Menu Plan for stubborn weight that starts on page 72. I've been amazed countless times at how resilient the human body can be. It doesn't matter how old you are or how far things may have slipped. Your body can almost always heal if given a chance. A few good recipes might be all the help it needs.

Don't feel overwhelmed by your symptoms, but do try to keep track of how you're feeling. Even vague symptoms are important. They are signs that the body is working hard to maintain its balance. The endocrine system produces hormones that bring the body back to balance. We don't feel well when our hormones start to drift. You know how some days are better than others? We all have minor issues that come and go. These are normal signs that our bodies are fighting to regain balance. You know something is wrong when almost every day becomes a bad day. Symptoms let us know something is off before disease sets in.

Since hormones change as we move through the years, symptoms become more common with time. I used to think of aging as something that happened to people in their eighties. Now I know that everyone is aging, no matter how old they are. Our hormones must always adapt to cumulative daily changes. We all face traumas and illnesses. Women can face the additional transitions of pregnancy and menopause. Your hormones change as you age. They change and they change you.

Of course, every symptom is not a hormonal symptom. Health is more complicated than that. But hormonal symptoms are commonly ignored. People tell their doctors about these symptoms but rarely receive effective solutions. Hormonal imbalances cause such troublesome symptoms because hormones control so much. This includes how well we generate energy, burn calories, eliminate wastes, maintain a daily rhythm, and repair our tissues. The body makes over seventy main hormones. Once you consider that each has many by-products and metabolites, we're taking about a lot of moving parts. The table on page 20 lists a few of the main ones and the roles they play.

# Hormones and Their Functions in the Body

If it seems like hormones do everything, how do you know if your symptoms are hormonal?

| HORMONE | ORIGIN(S) | TASKS |
| --- | --- | --- |
| Androgens: DHEA, testosterone | Adrenal glands<br>Testicles | Growth<br>Muscle repair<br>Reproduction |
| Estrogens: estrone, estradiol, estriol | Adipose tissue<br>Adrenal glands<br>Ovaries<br>Placenta | Bone growth<br>Menstruation<br>Reproduction |
| Leptin | Adipose tissue | Hunger<br>Metabolic rate |
| Melatonin | Pineal gland | Circadian rhythm<br>Immune regulation |
| Pancreatic endocrine hormones: glucagon, insulin, somatostatin | Pancreas | Blood sugar regulation |
| Stress hormones: cortisol, cortisone, pregnenolone | Adrenal glands<br>Liver | Circadian rhythm<br>Glucose regulation<br>Inflammation |
| Thyroid hormones: T3 and T4 | Thyroid gland | Basal metabolic rate<br>Keratin repair<br>Nerve conduction |

# Hormonal Symptoms

Since hormones regulate every facet of the body's chemistry, they can cause almost any symptom imaginable. But some are more typical than others. Some of the most common symptoms that point toward a hormone imbalance include:

- Weight gain
- Puffy face
- Muscle aches
- Insomnia
- Fatigue
- Thinning hair
- Depression
- Poor libido
- Hot flashes
- Cold sensitivity
- Anxiety
- Stretch marks
- Abnormal hunger
- Fat growth on the back
- Dark discolorations of the skin

Those are many of the possible ones. The problem with a list this long is that no one will have all of them, but nearly everyone will have some of them. It turns out that some symptoms are more predictive than others.

# The Most Significant Symptoms of a Hormone Imbalance

Over the years, I've shared online surveys with hundreds of thousands of people, asking which symptoms are most troublesome. Five symptoms keep coming up again and again because people with a hormone imbalance always have at least one of them:

- Weight gain
- Brain fog
- Fatigue
- Insomnia
- Hot flashes

Any one of these by itself can be a big deal, causing angst and grief. It can get in the way of your goals and block you from the life you know you deserve. One symptom can be a real problem, but most people with imbalanced hormones experience more than one. Many even have all five symptoms.

## WEIGHT GAIN

In every survey I've done, weight gain is the number one symptom by a lot. It is the most common complaint. The other characteristic of weight gain is that it can do the most to worsen the other symptoms. Extra weight can make you tired. Heavier women often have worse hot flashes. Weight gain can worsen memory. Belly fat can make it hard to breathe at night, contributing to poorer sleep quality.

I believe that much of the medicalization of body weight is not productive, but healthy habits lead to lower risks, even if they don't translate into weight loss. Weight loss is hard, and many may fail despite repeated attempts, but it's still worth trying to achieve if it can improve your quality of life.

All these symptoms can connect with one another, but weight gain is the hub. If your weight is one of the symptoms you're struggling with, it's the best place to get started. You can read more about possible culprits behind weight gain, effective strategies, meal plans, and recipes in chapters 3, 8, and 9.

## FATIGUE

We all get tired sometimes, but for some people, *sometimes* starts to feel more like all the time. A common pattern is for the normal afternoon slump to get worse, start earlier, and last longer. You might find yourself turning more to caffeine or sweets to boost your energy when you really need it.

Medically, fatigue is often not addressed if a clear cause is not found. If it lasts over six months and is so bad that it prevents more than half of your activities, it may be labeled as chronic fatigue syndrome. Receiving this diagnosis might give you the option of medical disability, but it does nothing to open up treatment options.

Fatigue can also worsen weight gain because it's harder to stay active. It can also lower mood by depriving you of essential things like exercise and socialization. You can read more about possible causes of fatigue, nutraceutical strategies, meal plans, and recipes in chapters 4, 8, and 9.

## HOT FLASHES

How do you know if you're having hot flashes? They say if you're in love, you know it. Hot flashes are kind of like that. If you have them, you know it. They typically last anywhere from several seconds to a few minutes. During this time your skin feels like it is on fire, your face and neck might flush, and you might break out in a sweat. Basically, imbalances in estrogen confuse your body's thermostat.

Hot flashes are bad enough at any time of day. When they happen at night, they can ruin your sleep. We refer to these as night sweats. They can also lead to ongoing anxiety, because you never know when they will come on next. Of course, night sweats can be a big contributor to sleep issues.

Hot flashes can be signs of deeper medical issues such as chronic infections or malignancies. But if you are a woman in your late thirties to mid-fifties, hot flashes do not necessarily mean there is something else wrong.

If you are of another age or gender and have severe hot flashes, talk to your doctor to see what the issue might be.

You can read more about effective strategies for hot flashes as well as meal plans and recipes in chapters 6, 8, and 9.

## BRAIN FOG

Sure, we all forget our keys on occasion. But it is unsettling when memory seems to fail more often. The lost keys, forgotten names, and missed appointments are all signs that something could be wrong. It is worth paying attention if it seems like little lapses are happening all the time.

Brain fog is common in those who are anemic, have thyroid disease, or have unstable blood sugar. It can also be the side effect of several medications. Talk to your doctor about brain fog and be sure to mention if it came on after starting on any new medication. Our brain and our muscles use energy in similar ways. Brain fog and fatigue often go together. Brain fog can often be a consequence of poor sleep or extra weight.

You can read more about effective strategies for brain fog as well as meal plans and recipes in chapters 5, 8, and 9.

## INSOMNIA

This symptom can include many variations—difficulty falling asleep, difficulty staying asleep, or unrefreshing sleep. You can't live well if you can't sleep well. You are edgier and more short-tempered. You won't recover as well from exercise. Your body won't be able to manage your blood sugar as well.

Poor sleep can directly worsen weight gain, fatigue, and brain fog. You can read more about strategies for insomnia as well as meal plans and recipes in chapters 7, 8, and 9.

---

*As bad as these symptoms can be, please know that food can be a solution. Our bodies depend on phytonutrients from food to maintain hormonal balance. These recipes will help you to use food strategically to regain your balance. The health you want might be just a few tasty meals away.*

---

You have access to the book's resources page as well. It has things like cooking videos with me, printable shopping lists, guides to nutraceuticals, and more. You can find it at www.hormonehealingcookbook.com /resources.

# Medical Conditions That May Disrupt Hormones

Along with aging and routine stressors, hormones can be disrupted by certain medical conditions. It is good to be aware of them because if ignored, they can stand in the way of your progress. Here are a few to keep in mind.

## ADRENAL STRESS

The misnomer *adrenal fatigue* has been used since the mid-1990s. In efforts to correct the misnomer, the conventional medical world has overreached and failed to recognize a real phenomenon. The condition is called hypothalamic-pituitary-adrenal (HPA) axis dysfunction. The hypothalamus, pituitary, and adrenals play a central role in the body's stress response, and collectively they are known as the HPA axis.

When chronic stress is too prolonged and significant, the HPA axis becomes maladapted, with a hair-trigger response. Minor stressors provoke it in ways that would normally be reserved for major stressors. It also becomes less able to shut down their stress response and allow the body to go into the parasympathetic state of repair. This condition can worsen almost any existing symptom and raise the risk of early death and most chronic diseases.

Hypothalamic-pituitary-adrenal stress has also been called simply adrenal stress. It usually manifests itself in erratic energy levels, especially when they worsen or improve at set times of the day. Energy levels can also correlate with symptoms of poor sleep and weight gain in the mid-body. As I mentioned above, while the term *adrenal fatigue* is often used, people with chronic stress often have *low* adrenal function. Stress doesn't "wear out" your adrenals, but it does cause your body to put them in time-out.

The body can deliberately slow down the adrenals to give itself a chance to heal. It might sound like a subtle distinction, but those who think your adrenals are fatigued often prescribe pills containing cortisol or try to raise your levels of cortisol with other treatments. If you take into account the misunderstanding involved, this makes sense, but unfortunately such treatment simply gives the body more of what it is trying to get a break from.

For those who have been diagnosed as having severe adrenal stress, the strategies in my book *The Adrenal Reset Diet* can be helpful. Many people can reverse the condition within just a few months.

## EARLY FATTY LIVER

Fatty liver disease may be the most common condition that no one knows of. The vast majority of those with weight issues likely have it, and only the smallest percent have ever received a diagnosis. When fat builds up in the liver, it can easily disrupt your hormone balance long before it is bad enough to warrant a diagnosis. Suspect early fatty liver whenever your waist circumference is equal to or greater than half of your height.

Early fatty liver disease can also dramatically slow metabolism. The good news is that liver diseases can be among the most reversible conditions. Those who suspect they have it can consider working through the process in *The Metabolism Reset Diet*.

## SUBOPTIMAL THYROID FUNCTION

Like most conditions, thyroid function exists along a continuum. There are many who do not have overt thyroid disease but also do not have optimal thyroid function. In such cases, the change in thyroid function can contribute to many symptoms, the top ones being weight gain, fatigue, and hair loss.

Recent studies have shown that 80 percent or more of overt thyroid disease can be reversed through diet. Those with milder forms of thyroid dysfunction have an even greater chance of recovery. Much of the solution hinges on the curious relationship between the thyroid gland and the mineral iodine. It turns out that there is a narrow range of iodine that may reverse stress on the thyroid. *The Thyroid Reset Diet* is a resource for those who have or are concerned about thyroid disease. It provides dietary plans based upon the latest evidence of disease reversal.

# Recipes or Resets?

If you have or suspect one of the above conditions, should you start with this cookbook or one of my other books? You don't have to choose. This cookbook can be used to supplement the recipes for any of them. Each of those books has a 28-day plan for one specific goal: recovery from adrenal stress (*Adrenal Reset Diet*), repair of a slow metabolism and fatty liver (*Metabolism Reset Diet*), and reversal of thyroid disease (*Thyroid Reset Diet*). Those books all have their own recipes, but you can never have too many!

Just follow the appropriate book's program and add in the recipes from this one as you see fit. Most of these recipes work, as they are in all the programs. Some require minimal modification, but each recipe tells you if it does and how to do it. Once you complete the reset program in the book you are following, you can use these recipes in your maintenance plan, or if you have remaining symptoms, you can try one of the 14-Day Menu Plans in this cookbook to help them. However you choose to get started, the important thing to keep in mind is that you have the ability to improve your health through diet. These symptoms can keep people from fully living. But they don't have to.

Changing your diet is hard only if you must give up good food. It isn't hard when you are learning to make new recipes that you like even better than what you ate before.

# CHAPTER 2

# Food & Hormones

Our body has an elaborate system of hormones that regulates everything and keeps us in good health. If hormones do their job well, we feel great. Once they lose their ability to regulate, we run into trouble. I will help you ditch the symptoms and get your hormones back in balance.

So how do hormones do what they do, and why don't they always work? It is not too much of a stretch to think of hormones as flavoring ingredients in your blood. In this analogy, the combination of hormones creates a distinct flavor that your cells taste. Your brain has a tiny organ called the hypothalamus. It is the master chef that adjusts the flavor of your blood on a minute-by-minute basis. You could imagine that the hypothalamus has a spice pantry with hundreds of bottles. Rather than cinnamon, ginger, and oregano, these spices include hormones like thyroid hormones, estrogen, cortisol, glucagon, testosterone, insulin, melatonin, leptin, and progesterone.

Your hypothalamus monitors your body's chemistry and decides whether your cells need to start doing something they are not, stop doing what they are already doing, speed something up, or slow something down. It flavors your blood with hormones to keep them in balance. How does it all work? Imagine a Monday morning.

*Beep! Beep! Beep!* It is 5:30 A.M. You were fast asleep and minding your own business when suddenly the alarm went off. Your hypothalamus realizes that you need to turn on your body, so it coaxes your adrenal glands to release cortisol. This is called the cortisol awakening response, and it helps your body use your thyroid hormones. At 4:00 A.M., your thyroid released its main batch of T4 and T3 for the day. The surge of cortisol allows the thyroid hormones to cross into your cells and turn on their mitochondria to make energy. The cortisol awakening response will also shut down any melatonin from the pineal gland so you can stay awake. Because you were not ready to get up, that will take a few hours to help. In the meantime, you desperately need coffee.

Once the caffeine enters your system by six, it causes your pancreas to release glucagon, which dumps any stored sugar into your bloodstream, making you feel alert while the systems come online. The resistant starch you had in last night's potatoes is still preventing you from overreacting to this surge in blood sugar. Otherwise, the extra sugar could cause your pancreas to make too much insulin for the whole day, leaving you in fat storage mode. Your hypothalamus knows your stress levels have been high at work. On your way to the office at 7:30 A.M., it makes more DHEA than normal. The DHEA will work along with the polyphenols from the blueberries you ate to prevent the extra cortisol from damaging your brain cells.

That was just a tiny piece of the action over a few hours of a single day. If we could be more detailed, we would see that every minute of the day, all these hormones and foods constantly interact with one another. They do so whether we are intentional about it or not. Your body has many internal systems to regulate its hormones, but things can go wrong. Four main factors push hormones out of balance: stress, too much food, chronic diseases, and aging, three of which are described below. In chapter 3, we discuss why and how extra food disrupts hormone balance.

## Stress

People often assume that stress is caused by exterior circumstances: a difficult work environment, a tumultuous relationship, or an unsettled home life. These factors can cause stress, but they aren't the only ones. Anything that pushes our bodies out of balance can be a source of stress, including:

- Feeling too cold or too warm
- Delays in mealtimes
- Anxiety about health
- Changes to the sleep schedule
- Abnormal blood sugar
- Chronic pain
- Too little time outside
- Social isolation

Things like this add up and raise our total stress load. The more stressors we face at a given time, the greater our total load. We all have a finite ability to keep it together under stress. Past a certain point, we don't bounce back, we break. The closer we get to this point, the more symptoms show up. Stress cranks up cortisol production, which disrupts blood sugar and raises inflammation. Foods can reverse both effects and thereby lower the harm from stress. Specific ingredients in food, such as resistant starch in beans, stabilize blood sugar. Others, like polyphenols in spinach, lower inflammation.

The way you'll learn to combine foods

into meals will also help. I've built these meals around veggies, protein, and healthy carbs. Stable blood sugar levels are essential for hormone balance. If your blood sugar surges up too quickly or drops down too low, your body has to undergo hormonal contortions to make things right. Such dramatic corrections help, but they often have rebound effects that last for days.

Meals with lean protein, good carbs, and veggies provide glucose as part of a mixture that is slowly absorbed into your bloodstream. It prevents the highs and lows and keeps your body's metabolism running well. Fats are included, but they don't require as much attention, because the necessary amounts are easy to get. They find their way in just fine.

# Diseases

When things are out of balance, the body works to make them right, but this higher level of effort can be harmful. Take autoimmune thyroid disease as an example. The immune system recognizes malfunctioning thyroid cells and eats them up to make room for new cells. But too much iodine can confuse the immune system, leading it to damage healthy thyroid cells. A response that is normally helpful turns harmful.

Diabetes is the most common disease that directly alters hormone levels. Others include polycystic ovary syndrome, Addison's disease, and premature ovarian failure (primary ovarian insufficiency).

Good food can often prevent disease, and it may also cure it. Recent studies have proved that many forms of thyroid disease and diabetes can be reversed with diet. Those might seem to be large claims, but they are backed up with strong evidence. In one study, diet alone reversed diabetes in 72 percent of participants within eight weeks.[1] CT scans showed that their pancreases had physically changed, and the disease was no longer present. Three months later, the results still held. In another study, a dietary intervention was tested with people who'd had severe thyroid disease for four years on average but were not taking thyroid medication. Within three months of diet therapy, 78.3 percent of them were found to have perfectly normal thyroid function.[2]

# Normal Aging

All hormone levels change with age, some more than others. Men and women in their sixties have much less estrogen and testosterone than men and women in their thirties. If the change is gradual, we can adapt and not notice it, but sometimes the transition is rapid. Erratic swings in hormones can lead to hot flashes, fatigue, and insomnia. As hormone levels become imbalanced, we become less resilient. Good health is still possible, but it becomes harder to take it for granted.

Most people can coast along with little concern for their health until their forties or fifties. But somewhere around this point, they become either perpetual patients or health nuts. Both types are likely to face medical episodes like illness or surgeries, which involve risk. Those with less resilience are more likely to develop complications. Diagnoses and medications start to stack up. Soon life becomes a long series of visits to the doctor.

Chronic diseases can shorten our lifespan by several years. An even more dramatic difference is the quality of the last decades of life. Many of us lose our ability to enjoy the most basic things like a walk outside, a good meal, or the ability to be present with our loved ones. Our lifespan is how long we live. Our "healthspan" is how much we live.

The other path is that of the health nut. They treat health like a hobby. They enjoy spending time on recreational exercise, cooking, and health education. Health nuts may live a few years longer. But their healthspan may be decades longer. Studies have shown that the healthiest of the elderly live as well as those who are thirty to forty years younger! So how does food change this trajectory?

## How Food Helps Hormones

We rely on hormones, and so does our food. Plants make compounds to regulate their own hormones as well as those of other plants and insects. When we eat these compounds, in addition to vitamins, minerals, and protein, we do a better job at keeping our own hormones in balance.

### PHYTONUTRIENTS

Human nutrition is a surprisingly young science. Only within the last century or so were vitamins identified. It turned out that certain substances in food were necessary, and a complete lack of them could be fatal. These substances came to be called essential nutrients.

Some took this discovery to a seemingly logical conclusion, deciding that a diet could be defined as healthy or unhealthy solely on the presence of essential nutrients. A healthy diet supplied these nutrients, an unhealthy one did not, and no other variables were relevant. If this idea had been true, anyone on a junk food diet who took a basic multivitamin would be just as healthy as anyone else. Yet we know that is not the case.

Nutrition scientists agree that minimally processed plant foods are teeming with compounds that improve our health, even if they aren't necessarily deemed essential. Such compounds are known as phytonutrients. Here are a couple of the main categories of phytonutrients and their health benefits.

## Carotenoids

Carotenoids are colorful pigments found in a wide range of fruits and vegetables. They work to neutralize free radicals and protect cells from damage. Studies have shown that diets rich in carotenoids lower the risk for macular degeneration. Carotenoids also lower the odds of lung and colorectal cancer.

## Sulfur Compounds

The element sulfur is an essential component of collagen and keratin. As such, diets rich in sulfur compounds correlate with healthier hair, skin, and nails. Sulfur compounds are also used in liver reactions that eliminate hormone by-products, thus keeping hormones in a state of healthy balance.

## Phenolics

Compounds with aromatic rings and hydroxyl groups are known as phenolics. The word *aromatic* has a more sciency meaning here, but the everyday meaning still applies. Phenolics do contribute to the aroma and flavor of foods. Plants make phenolics to protect themselves against UV damage, predators, and infections. When we eat them, they help us in much the same ways. They also play roles in the regulation of our hormones and blood sugar.

## Phytosterols

*Phyto* means "plant," and *sterol* refers to a hormone built from a sterol ring. Our sterol hormones include all hormones from the adrenals, ovaries, and testicles. Phytosterols are similar enough to our sterols that they help our bodies make better use of them. Diets rich in phytosterols help our bodies make appropriate amounts of sterols, direct them to the most helpful cell receptors, and break them down effectively with fewer harmful by-products. This is how we balance our hormones.

Recent high-quality studies have shown that diets highest in these phytonutrients help us live longer and feel better. They regulate hormones, cut the risk of chronic disease, help control body weight, and improve mental function.[3] Phytonutrients don't force your body to do more of something or less of something else. They help it control itself more effectively. And because phytonutrients help your body reach a state of balance, you don't even have to know which hormones are too high or too low. Food can still help. To choose the right recipes, all you need to know are which symptoms are the worst.

## Why Not Just Take Phytonutrients in Supplement Form?

It can be tempting to think that we can take the magic ingredient and put it into a pill. Some said onions were healthy because they contained quercetin. Yet studies showed that quercetin supplements did not do what onions could. Countless other studies show the same thing—food constituents are not food. Why is that the case?

Studying food constituents is helpful because it is easier. We can study these compounds in test tubes and animal models. Such preliminary research can be used to inspire larger human studies on food, but we cannot expect that phytonutrients in isolation will work exactly like food. When employed carefully, a reductionistic look can help us predict which foods are healthiest for us. But breaking food down into its constituent parts still does not confer the same benefits as eating the food itself.

Not only are whole foods better than food fractions, but I strongly believe that simple everyday foods are better than exotic superfoods. My top picks are foods you have already heard of and know where to find. Along with onions, some of my favorite ingredients include oats, carrots, spinach, garlic, figs, and oranges. The recipes are organized by the top five symptoms of hormone imbalance: weight gain, fatigue, brain fog, hot flashes, and insomnia. Each symptom has its own two-week menu plan that focuses on the top recipe for that symptom.

You can choose recipes that sound good or choose a two-week plan to prioritize a particular symptom.

| CATEGORY | CAROTENOIDS | SULFUR COMPOUNDS |
|---|---|---|
| EXAMPLES | Alpha-carotene<br>Astaxanthin<br>Beta-carotene<br>Beta-cryptoxanthin<br>Lycopene<br>Lutein<br>Zeaxanthin | Allicin<br>Diallyl sulfide<br>Glucosinolates<br>Methylsulfonylmethane (MSM)<br>Sulforaphane<br>Thiosulfate |
| FOOD SOURCES | Cantaloupe<br>Carrots<br>Kale<br>Mangoes<br>Pumpkin<br>Shrimp<br>Spinach<br>Squash<br>Sweet potatoes<br>Tomatoes | Almonds<br>Broccoli<br>Brown rice<br>Brussels sprouts<br>Cabbage<br>Cauliflower<br>Garlic<br>Leeks<br>Lentils<br>Oats<br>Onions |
| BENEFITS | Lower cancer risk<br>Improve eye health | Heal connective tissues<br>Regulate hormones |

# Phytonutrients

| PHENOLICS | PHYTOSTEROLS | OTHERS |
|---|---|---|
| Curcumin | Beta-sitosterol | Capsaicin |
| Epigallocatechin gallate (EGCG) | Campesterol | Essential fats |
| Flavonoids | Stanols | Nitrates |
| Gallic acid | Stigmasterol | Melatonin |
| Lignans | | Resistant starch |
| Proanthocyanins | | |
| Resveratrol | | |
| Tannic acid | | |
| | | |
| Basil | Cashews | Cayenne |
| Black olives | Canola oil | Sunflower seeds |
| Capers | Flaxseed | Beets |
| Celery seed | Pistachios | Pistachios |
| Cloves | Rye flour | Potatoes |
| Currants | Sesame seeds | |
| Ginger | Walnuts | |
| Oregano | Wheat germ | |
| Peppermint | Whole wheat | |
| Raspberries | | |
| Rosemary | | |
| Tea | | |
| | | |
| Lower inflammation | Lower cholesterol | Boost metabolism |
| Improve circulation | Prevent heart disease | Improve gut flora |
| Regulate blood sugar | | Increase tissue oxygen |

# Your First 2 Weeks

If you have several symptoms, how should you start?
Here is a quick quiz that will help you decide.
It should take less than two minutes to complete.

## HORMONE IMBALANCE QUIZ

Answer each question yes or no. Total the number of yes answers
for each section.

### SECTION A

1. My weight has changed dramatically in the last few years. Y/N

2. I often eat more than I plan to. Y/N

3. Eating healthy doesn't help me lose weight. Y/N

4. Given how little I eat, I should not weigh what I do. Y/N

5. I exercise more than my friends, but they are thinner. Y/N

**TOTAL NUMBER OF YES ANSWERS** ____

### SECTION B

1. I need coffee more than I ever used to. Y/N

2. By evening I'm too exhausted to do anything useful. Y/N

3. If I try to do everything I should, I'll be wiped out for days. Y/N

4. I avoid social events because I don't have the energy. Y/N

5. My favorite days are ones in which I can rest as much as I want. Y/N

**TOTAL NUMBER OF YES ANSWERS** ____

## SECTION C

1. My periods have stopped or become unpredictable.    Y/N

2. I often feel full or bloated.    Y/N

3. Sometimes my breasts feel lumpy or tender.    Y/N

4. I suffer from hot flashes.    Y/N

5. My sex drive is low or unpredictable.    Y/N

**TOTAL NUMBER OF YES ANSWERS** ____

## SECTION D

1. I struggle with remembering first names.    Y/N

2. I make more lists and notes because I'm afraid of forgetting things.    Y/N

3. Sometimes I walk into a room and forget why I went there.    Y/N

4. My loved ones tell me I repeat myself more.    Y/N

5. I keep losing my keys or my phone.    Y/N

**TOTAL NUMBER OF YES ANSWERS** ____

## SECTION E

1. It takes too long to get to sleep.    Y/N

2. I wake up in the middle of the night and can't get back to sleep.    Y/N

3. Even if I get enough sleep, it feels less refreshing.    Y/N

4. If I sit still in the afternoon, I'll probably fall asleep.    Y/N

5. As soon as I lie down to sleep, my mind starts racing.    Y/N

**TOTAL NUMBER OF YES ANSWERS** ____

| SECTION | SYMPTOM | YOUR SCORE |
|---------|---------|------------|
| A | Weight | |
| B | Fatigue | |
| C | Hot flashes | |
| D | Brain fog | |
| E | Sleep | |

## Where to start?

- If one section's score was the highest, start with that symptom.

- If several scores tie, choose the one you've had the longest.

- If all five scores are high, start with weight.

If you do have several symptoms with scores of 3 or greater, repeat the quiz after your first two-week challenge. Your symptoms may have changed, and some symptoms will have improved more than others. Your new score may direct you to a new challenge or suggest that you should repeat the last one. Stubborn symptoms may continue to improve with several challenges. When you start a new challenge or repeat the last one, you can start the two-week plan right away. It is not necessary to take a break before starting one.

In the next section, I will devote a chapter to each of the main symptoms: weight, fatigue, brain fog, hot flashes, and insomnia. In each chapter, I'll explain more about what this symptom looks like, and how it happens in the body. I'll explore which foods can help each symptom, and how they work.

Because it is the one symptom that is the biggest driver of the other symptoms, we will start with weight.

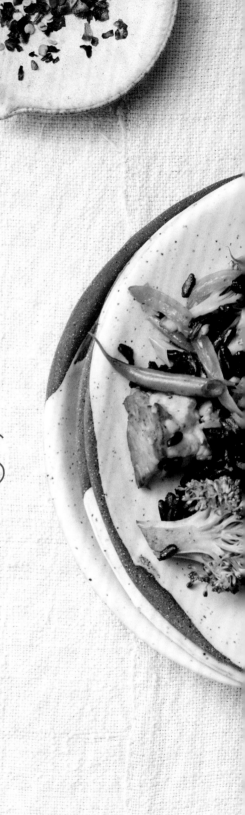

PART 2

# SPECIFIC
# SYMPTOMS

# CHAPTER 3

# Weight

We talk about weight as the main issue, but the real problem is fat—especially fat in the wrong places. I wish we could banish the word *fat* and start over.

I say that for two reasons. First, the word itself has inflicted too much emotional pain. Second, it refers to so many different things. The word *fat* might refer to the adipose cells in our bodies, to dietary nutrients also known as lipids, or to energy-carrying triglycerides in our bloodstream.

Fat in itself is not bad. In fact, it is essential to our health. We need fat in our diets and some fat in our bodies. But too much fat can cause ongoing symptoms and shorten your lifespan. How would you know if you have too much? The simplest way is to calculate your waist-to-height ratio. Take the number of inches around your waist and divide it by your height. If your answer is greater than 0.5, you may have unsafe amounts of fat.

Here is a quick example: Imagine that a 5'5" woman has a 30-inch waist circumference (5'5" = 65 inches, and 30 ÷ 65 = 0.46). She's okay. Now imagine a 5'9" man with a 36-inch waist: 5'9" = 69 inches, and 36 ÷ 69 = 0.52. That's too high. Extra fat is a risk unto its own even when other factors like blood pressure, blood sugar, and cholesterol are healthy. It is a risk for early death from all causes, including heart disease, cancers, and stroke. It also correlates with risks for gallbladder disease, osteoarthritis, liver disease, brain aging, fatty liver, and disability.

Please know that even tiny reductions in fat can improve all these things. Most of the health benefits show up from losing the first few pounds. In fact, reducing just 1 gram of extra fat from the organs can reverse type 2 diabetes![1] One gram is about the mass of a paper clip. Fat loss does not have to be major to be majorly helpful.

---

*Fat can refer to a large range of lipids in the diet. Butter, lard, fish oil, Crisco, canola oil, palm oil, avocados—these are all distinct, but they are all called fats. Fat can also refer to circulating fuel in the form of triglycerides or cholesterol. Even below the skin, there are many kinds of body fat. Some types burn fuel, some store it. Some improve health, some generate inflammation. Body fat can even change from good types to bad types or vice versa.*

Even the word *fat* itself is complicated. It has long been a derogatory label.

Our society often posits unrealistic expectations regarding how much weight someone can lose and how easy it is to do so. Weight loss is not easy, and radical, lasting weight loss is not the norm. Weight loss is hard in the best of circumstances, but a hormone imbalance makes it even harder. When a person's hormones are off, the body can be locked in a storage mode and fat stays locked in place.

Nonetheless, it is possible to lose enough weight to feel better. Even though it is not easy, weight loss is possible and there are valid reasons to pursue it. How common is this issue? Studies suggest that more than 85 percent of adults are *overfat*. This is a new term that denotes both those who are heavier than ideal and those who are at a healthy weight but have too much fat and too little muscle.

Our modern culture does not help. All too often, people have a hard time accessing whole foods or finding the means to exercise. These dilemmas make the stress of extra weight that much more acute. In addition to its emotional toll and health risks, extra fat can be behind many ongoing symptoms.

## Weight-Related Symptoms

The health risks of obesity are well understood. Most know about the increase in overall mortality, diabetes, heart disease, arthritis, and many cancers. But many are surprised to know that extra weight can be the source of many troublesome symptoms. If you don't feel good about your weight, consider any chronic symptoms as one more motivation to try a new approach.

## Finding the Cause

There are many medical conditions that make weight gain more likely. Thyroid disease is the biggest culprit of hormone imbalance that leads to weight gain, and it has the most dramatic effects. It can slow the metabolic rate by 60 percent. Others include sleep apnea, polycystic ovary syndrome (PCOS), and Cushing's disease. If it seems like you're stuck, ask your doctor if any of these or other conditions could be behind it.

Medications can also be an issue. Antidepressants, diabetic medications, oral contraceptives, and steroids are well-known contributors. Has weight been a bigger issue after starting a new medication? If so, ask your doctor if other options are available.

# How Specific Foods Can Help

The right foods can help maintain fat loss. Certain foods can boost your metabolism rate, helping you burn calories more quickly. Others can help you fill up more quickly, making you naturally eat less. Some foods cause you to absorb fewer calories. Foods can also improve inflammation levels, helping you send more energy to muscle tissue and less to fat. The foods that follow have been proven to work in one or more of these ways.

For each food, I'll share some of the evidence behind why I chose it. In most cases, clinical trials showed that frequent use of the food led to weight loss. Because these foods help with the same goal, you don't have to eat any one of them every day. By following the 14-Day Menu Plan, you'll get several helpful ingredients each day.

## CAYENNE

Cayenne pepper, the powdered fruit taken from the cayenne pepper plant, is a common spice used in cooking. It imparts a hot or spicy flavor into dishes. How does cayenne help manage weight? Many of its effects stem from an alkaloid called capsaicin. This alkaloid stimulates the sympathetic nervous system to raise the body's heat production. Once the body's thermostat goes up, several helpful processes occur:[2]

- Reduced appetite, increased satiety

- Better burning of fat as fuel

- Increased thermogenesis (causes the body to burn more fuel)

- Inhibited lipase and alpha-amylase (prevents the absorption of calories)

- Prevention of the development of new fat cells

Compared to those on the placebo, those taking cayenne lost more body fat, burned more calories, and had more improvements of blood sugar regulation.[3] What if you can't eat spicy foods? Thankfully you're still in luck, because even small amounts of cayenne can help. It can also be used in supplement form.

## POTATOES

Potatoes, a fat-loss food! Really!? If you're not eating them in the form of French fries or potato chips, yes, potatoes deserve their place on this list.

A few years ago, the director of the Washington State Potato Commission was frustrated about the bad rap potatoes were getting during the peak of the low-carb craze. He decided to go public with himself as a test case to prove that potatoes could be healthy. For sixty days, he ate nothing but potatoes—about twenty per day. If the Atkins ideas about carbs, insulin, and weight had been correct, he should have become heavier than ever. He did not. Over the sixty days, he lost 21 pounds and lowered his cholesterol levels by 67 points.[4]

Diets high in resistant starch reduce belly fat, lower insulin, and improve weight loss. When boiled or steamed, potatoes are the highest known source of resistant starch. They have more potassium than bananas, and plenty of vitamin C. Besides their resistant starch, potatoes help fat loss because they are filling. Calorie per calorie, potatoes lower the appetite more effectively than any other food.

In a study, a large group of adults were given controlled servings of a single specific test food after an overnight fast. Each serving was adjusted to provide the same number of calories regardless of the food. Before and after eating, the participants rated their hunger scores. After the participants had eaten, researchers tracked how long they waited to eat again and how much they had in the follow-up meal. If a food was more filling than another, an equal size serving of it would fill people up longer and cause them to eat less afterward. In all, 43 foods were tested. Based on the results, each food was assigned a satiety score. The foods that filled people up the longest were given higher scores. Those that left people hungrier were given lower scores.

## Most Filling Foods

| FOOD | SATIETY SCORE |
|---|---|
| Potatoes | 323 |
| Codfish | 225 |
| Oatmeal | 209 |
| Oranges | 202 |
| Apples | 197 |
| Whole grain pasta | 188 |

## Least Filling Foods

| FOOD | SATIETY SCORE |
|---|---|
| Croissants | 47 |
| Cake | 65 |
| Doughnuts | 68 |
| Candy bar | 70 |
| Peanuts | 84 |

With a score of 323, potatoes were in a class by themselves! No other food had even close to the same effect on satiety. The study used boiled potatoes seasoned with salt.[5]

The more your diet contains high-satiety foods, the more you fill up and the less you eat. No single food can achieve these goals better than potatoes.

## GINGER

Ginger, the common culinary spice, has a large body of evidence attesting to its benefits on body fat. It is rich in polyphenols, including 6-gingerol, 8-gingerol, and 10-gingerol. These compounds enter the liver through the portal veins and have been shown to increase thermogenesis, decrease the buildup of liver fat, improve insulin sensitivity, and improve the brain's regulation of hunger.[6]

In a double-blind placebo-controlled study, 80 obese women were given capsules of powdered ginger or a placebo for 12 weeks. Compared with the placebo group, those taking ginger saw a dramatic decrease in their body mass index scores and a reduction in body fat.[7] Other studies have confirmed this effect and proven that regular use of ginger can cause decreases in hip and waist circumference.[8]

You'll find ginger in many of these recipes. Regular use of ginger tea is another easy way to add it to your diet.

## ONIONS

Could onions help you lose belly fat? Belly fat, otherwise known as visceral fat, is a killer. When there is too much belly fat, it can start building up inside the liver and the pancreas, leading to diabetes. Animal studies suggest that the plant pigment quercetin may reduce the formation of belly fat. Yet no studies confirmed this effect on humans.

Because of this information, a group of scientists was inspired to see if quercetin-rich foods could help human volunteers shed belly fat. They chose onions in the form of onion powder as the source of quercetin. The participants all got roughly 1 tablespoon of onion powder daily. Those on the placebo group got a low-quercetin version, while the active group got high-quercetin onion powder. Neither group was asked to change their diets, and both were tracked for 12 weeks.

The total abdominal fat went down dramatically in those on high-quercetin onion powder. Couldn't you just take a pill of quercetin and get the same results? Probably not. The results were more about onions than about quercetin. It turned out that even low-quercetin onions still helped.[9] Onion skins contain massive amounts of phytonutrients. Try to save them for adding to soups and stocks. Onion Skin Rice, one of the recipes you'll find in this book, makes use of onion skins to boost the phytonutrient content of rice (page 163).

# Nutraceutical Solutions

## CHOLINE

Choline is an essential nutrient required to convert dietary fats into energy. Many individuals cannot adequately synthesize choline, and many diets are lacking in it. In a double-blind human clinical trial, women were given supplements with choline or a placebo for seven days. None were instructed to undergo dietary modifications. Compared with those on the placebo, those taking choline had lower leptin levels and saw a 3 percent reduction in body fat. These changes came without the loss in performance typical of weight loss.[10]

## NIGELLA SATIVA

*Nigella sativa*, also known as black cumin, is a culinary seed. It has been used for thousands of years as a traditional medicine and a source of cooking oil in the Middle East. It has anti-inflammatory and immune-regulating properties. Since it has a long history of use as a food, nigella is considered safe for general usage over a wide range of dosages. Evidence shows that nigella helps weight loss through an improved breakdown of liver fat and an increase in insulin sensitivity by muscle cells. It also may act as a lipase inhibitor, lowering the absorption of fat from the diet.

In a recent clinical trial, people with thyroid disease were randomly distributed to receive a supplement containing either nigella or a placebo. Those receiving nigella saw significant improvements in body weight, body mass index, waist circumference, and hip circumference.[11]

## WHITE KIDNEY BEAN EXTRACT

White kidney beans (*Phaseolus vulgaris*) are like the common cannellini bean and are a rich source of resistant starch. Extracts of white kidney beans have been shown to slow the absorption of carbohydrates into the bloodstream. A recent review of multiple clinical trials on white kidney bean extract (WKBE) showed that it has caused weight loss in numerous clinical trials.[12]

The extract appears to help by lowering the activity of the enzyme amylase, which breaks complex carbohydrates into simple carbohydrates. It also reduces the rate at which carbohydrates leave the stomach and enter the small intestines. WKBE also improves the gut microbiota. Some of these improvements have direct benefits to weight management, while others can help in the recovery from autoimmune diseases.

*To learn more about how to use these and other nutraceutical ingredients, please visit the resources page at www.hormonehealing cookbook.com/resources.*

CHAPTER 4

# Fatigue

Do you ever find yourself feeling tired for no reason? If so, you're not alone. At any given point in time, up to 20 percent of perfectly healthy people can complain of fatigue. A recent survey of American adults found that the average woman feels unusually tired three or more days each week![1]

Fatigue is one of the single most common complaints in all of medicine. By some estimates, it is the cause of up to 20 percent of medical visits.[2] Despite how frequently the condition occurs, medicine doesn't have any good solutions for it. Fatigue can be caused by almost anything or nothing at all; there are no ways to measure it and no effective treatments. If anything, fatigue is likely underreported. People living with fatigue over the long term become resigned to it, rather than trying to improve their symptoms.

It is not easy to define fatigue. Biomedical researchers define it as "unusual overwhelming tiredness that is not comparable to physiologic exhaustion after physical or mental effort and which cannot be recovered by restful sleep."[3] In other words, tiredness can be expected, especially after unusual effort. Yet we expect it to go away with rest. When we are tired without exerting any unusual effort and no amount of rest helps, we call it fatigue.

Like most symptoms of a hormone imbalance, fatigue is usually found in conjunction with other symptoms. When you're tired, you're tired in lots of ways—physical, mental, or most commonly both. Many who have had fatigue for some time have become resigned to it. But fatigue can be dangerous to ignore. The EPIC-Norfolk study is an ongoing study of over 30,000 people who have been carefully tracked since 1993. Those who were the most tired had up to an 89 percent higher risk of early death, a figure that still stood even after medical conditions were factored in. Unresolved fatigue is more than just a nuisance.[4]

These participants experienced fatigue in a variety of ways. Most at risk for disease were those whose fatigue prevented them from exercising. When surveyed, most adults say they would exercise more if they had more energy.

# Causes of Fatigue

Most fatigue is unexplained, yet sometimes there is a specific cause. It's worth trying to find the cause, because improvement can be unlikely unless you know what you're treating. Some of the common conditions to consider include:

- Anemia
- $B_{12}$ deficiency
- Depression and anxiety
- Obesity
- Parathyroid disease
- Psychosocial stress
- Sleep apnea, insomnia
- Thyroid disease

How do you know if you have any of these? A good diagnostician can talk you through the possibilities and gather some data from a physical exam. Based on how you respond, they may use symptom surveys to check for anxiety, depression, and psychosocial stress; blood tests for anemias, $B_{12}$ levels, and thyroid disease; and a sleep study if sleep apnea seems suspicious.

If a cause can't be found, that does not mean your symptoms are not real. They are, and the recipes in this book can still help your body produce energy more effectively. If a cause can be found, please follow through with suggested treatments and know that these recipes can help your treatments give you results more quickly.

# Eating for Energy

Time for some positive news about fatigue. We have good evidence that the right foods can still be helpful, regardless of the cause of fatigue. Those foods rich in the right constituents aid each cell's mitochondria in forming the adenosine triphosphate (ATP) that powers our bodies. Foods supply the fuel that mitochondria run on, and the right foods have phytonutrients that help the mitochondrial pathways run smoothly.

Since there is no blood test for fatigue, most studies rely on survey data. Surveys have been used on people with fatigue from causes such as thyroid disease, acute infections, cardiovascular disease, stroke, or cancer. The surveys get a baseline fatigue score for people known to be at risk for fatigue. Then the researchers have them add a specific food into their diets for a prescribed period, after which they repeat the survey.

The other large source of information has been endurance athletes. In these cases, fatigue is expected, yet it is often driven by the same biochemical mechanisms that cause fatigue in cases of illness. With athletes, the results are easy to measure. If a food lowers their fatigue, performance goes up. They become able to push harder, last longer, or go faster.

An encouraging finding from these studies is that quite often a food that improves fatigue from one cause also works to improve it when the cause is completely different.

In the rest of this chapter, I'll tell you about which foods can help you regain your energy. You'll be happy to see that all our top picks are easy to find and cook with.

# Foods for Energy

## ALMONDS

Almonds are dense sources of many nutrients and helpful phytochemicals, including vitamin E, magnesium, copper, and arginine. These nutrients are known to improve energy by lowering inflammation, improving the activity of muscle cells, and helping oxygen reach the tissues more effectively.

Like other unprocessed foods, almonds are more than the sum of their parts. In a study to test this idea, almonds were compared to cookies that provided the same calories and roughly the same amount of fat, carbohydrate, and protein. Trained endurance athletes added either the almonds or the cookies to their diets for four weeks and switched to the other for the following four weeks. Even though the foods were carefully matched in calories and fat, the almonds showed clear performance benefits that the cookies did not. Cyclists eating almonds were able to ride over half a mile farther during a timed trial while requiring less oxygen.[5]

## BEETS

Beets are in a class by themselves as the leading fatigue-fighting food. Athletes have known this for some time and embraced beets in a variety of forms. Among many endurance athletes, a shot of beet juice is as important before a race as tying their shoes.

### Nitrates and Oxygen

The story of beets and energy depends on a basic understanding of nitrates. Nitrates are nitrogen-containing compounds found in many foods. Nitrates occur naturally in some foods and are added to other foods as preservatives.

The main sources of natural nitrates include beets and greens. Nitrate-based preservatives are found mostly in processed meat like bacon and sausages. Nitrates give us a good teaching example of food being more than the sum of its parts. Even though the chemical form of nitrates is the same in all these foods, the health effects are the exact opposite.

It turns out that the food context changes how nitrates act. In processed meats, nitrates are combined with saturated fats and cooked at high heat. In vegetables, nitrates are found within a wide range of antioxidants and fibers. The consensus is that nitrates from vegetables are safe and enhance energy levels, while the same nitrates from processed meat can be harmful. Studies have shown that nitrates from vegetables lower the risk of stomach cancer, whereas the same nitrates from bacon raise the risk of stomach cancer.[6]

Beets and nitrates help us produce nitrous oxide. When oxygen levels dip, blood cells make nitrous oxide to help raise it. Nitrous oxide is also required to prevent hormone imbalances—it plays a role in regulating thyroid, ovarian, adrenal, and pituitary hormones. If your body can't make nitrous oxide well, beet juice can help. When your muscles use oxygen better, you have more energy, sharper cognition, and more graceful aging.

## Dietary Sources of Nitrate

Most vegetables provide some nitrate, but the amount varies tremendously among different types.[7]

The highest concentration of nitrate can be found among certain types of leafy greens like arugula or watercress. Beets are not as

## Nitrates in Foods

| NITRATE CONTENT (MG/100 G FRESH WEIGHT) | FOOD SOURCES |
| --- | --- |
| Very low, less than 20 mg | Artichoke, asparagus, broad bean, eggplant, garlic, green bean, mushroom, onion, pea, pepper, potato, summer squash, sweet potato, tomato, watermelon |
| Low, 20 to less than 50 mg | Broccoli, carrot, cauliflower, chicory, cucumber, pumpkin |
| Middle, 50 to less than 100 mg | Cabbage, dill, savoy cabbage, turnip |
| High, 100 to less than 250 mg | Celeriac, Chinese cabbage, endive, fennel, kohlrabi, leek, parsley |
| Very high, more than 250 mg | Arugula (rocket), chervil, cress, lettuce, red beets, spinach |

dense a source of nitrate as greens, but a typical serving size of beets is so much heavier that it yields more total nitrate.

Many studies have proven that beets boost energy and improve exercise performance. Some also show benefits to brain health. In one such study, two groups of adults in their mid-sixties were put on a gentle exercise regimen for six weeks. One set consumed beet juice; the other set did not. Both groups were given brain MRI scans. The group given beets showed greater signs of neuroplasticity—meaning that their brains benefited from the exercise more than expected.[8] Those consuming beets also became able to train at a higher intensity.

Many of these studies have been done on athletes, but similar results have been demonstrated in nonathletes. In fact, nonathletes may even see more dramatic benefits. For example, one study looked at the effects of beets on adults with fatigue from heart failure. The regular use of beets for just seven days increased aerobic endurance by 24 percent.[9]

## GARLIC

Garlic has a special place on our list because it has been shown to improve fatigue even when the cause is unknown.[10] The benefits

# LOW-CARB FATIGUE?

Are you getting enough good carbs? The human body can still generate energy on a low-carbohydrate diet, but not as much. Our main energy sources are fats and carbs. Fats have a greater energy density than carbohydrates, which have led some to think they are a superior source of fuel. When we dig deeper into the biochemistry, we learn that fats can't be burned effectively without carbohydrates.

A recent study showed that low-carb diets can make people tired. In the study, twenty-four women were put on a low-carb, high-fat diet for four weeks. Then for fifteen weeks, they were allowed to eat as they chose, followed by four more weeks on a diet that reduced food consumption without going low-carb. The second diet was meant to see if any negative symptoms from the low-carb diet were simply from less food, not fewer carbs.

On each diet, the researchers tracked the women's energy levels and measured how well they could exercise. Energy levels were tracked, with surveys about their daily symptoms, and participants kept a journal to document how they felt.

While on the low-carb diet, they reported that they felt "muscle fatigue, lactic acid in mus-

of garlic seem to be associated with numerous sulfur-containing phytonutrients such as allicin, diallyl sulfide (DAS), and S-allyl cysteine. Collectively these compounds are known to act as antioxidants, anti-inflammatories, immunomodulators, and neuroprotectants.

In a randomized double-blind, placebo-controlled study, seventy women with rheumatoid arthritis received either garlic or a placebo supplement for eight weeks. Those receiving garlic saw their fatigue scores decline by 14 percent on average. No such change was seen in the placebo group. Garlic also improved their pain levels and several markers of inflammation.[11] Garlic can also reverse fatigue secondary to chronic pain and autoimmune disease.

Garlic has been shown to combat brain fog. It can improve mental fatigue and even reduce the effects of aging on the brain.[12] It might be tempting to dismiss garlic, since most people eat garlic regularly. Yet when used in higher than typical amounts, it can do much to improve energy.

## OATS

Oats are a good source of low-glycemic carbohydrates and resistant starch, which means that they give you long periods of energy and steady blood sugar. Oats also boost energy

cles, and feeling tired." Several of them said that normal activities like going for walks or using the stairs were too difficult to complete.[13] Their exercise performance also suffered. When the women were on the low-carb diet, the level of exertion that was easy when eating carbs felt too hard. During tests on a stationary bike, the low-carb group became exhausted and had to stop pedaling over two minutes sooner.

If you feel tired and are on a low-carb diet, it's worth reconsidering adding more carbs. Carbs include a wide range of foods from Twinkies and sodas to tomatoes and black-eyed peas. It is silly to treat them all the same. Healthy carbs are the only foods that allow for a healthy microbial flora. Good bacteria cannot live without carbs.

Many people end up eating more protein when they go low-carb. Doing so can help boost energy and facilitate weight loss. But all the studies on low-carb diets that control for protein show that the benefits come from more protein, not fewer carbs.

If you've been low-carb for some time, I'd encourage you to see for yourself. Add back in some good healthy carbs like whole grains, beans, vegetables, and fruits, and see how you feel. If after two weeks, this diet does not help your fatigue, you can always go back. If you do feel better with carbs, please know that fat loss can work just fine without extreme deprivation. Look at chapter 3 on weight for more insights.

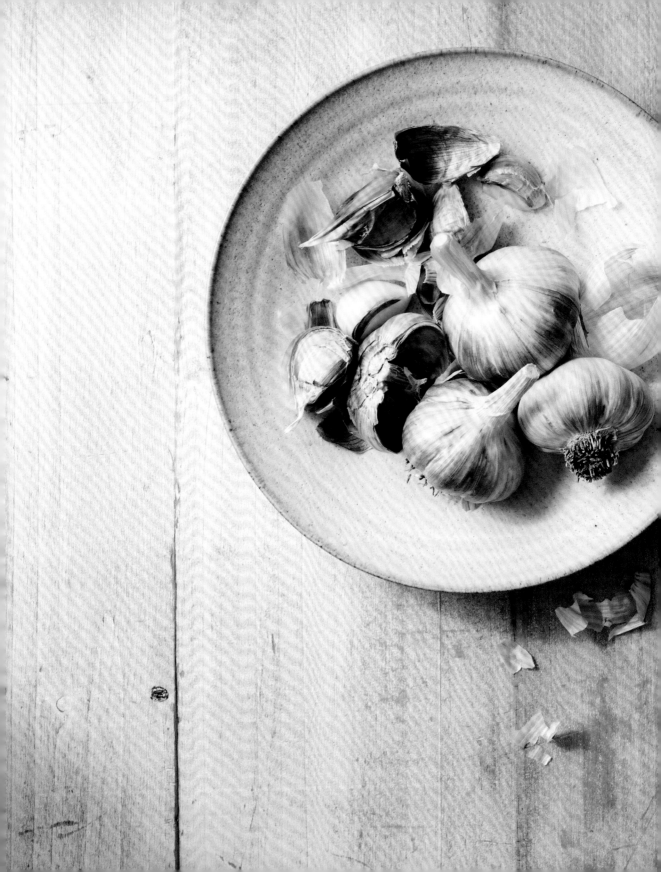

because they are one of the richest sources of a fatigue-fighting fiber called beta-glucan. A typical bowl of oatmeal contains as much as 2,000 mg of beta-glucan.

In a recent study on oats and fatigue, 207 adults were given oat beta-glucan and tracked over a four-week period. Compared with a control group, those consuming oats had lower scores on fatigue, exhaustion, and lack of energy. They also saw improvements in their ability to concentrate.[14] In addition to helping fatigue, oats have a large range of health benefits. They improve digestion, cardiovascular health, stress-related symptoms, and cognitive function.[15]

## WALNUTS

Walnuts have two advantages over other foods that make them powerful at fighting fatigue. The first is that they contain unique compounds called walnut oligopeptides. The second is that they are among the highest food sources of linoleic acid.

### Walnut Oligopeptides

Walnut oligopeptides are small chains of amino acids with unique properties. Studies show that walnut oligopeptides decrease the buildup of metabolic wastes such as lactate dehydrogenase, creatine kinase, blood urea nitrogen, and blood lactic acid. They also improve essential functions such as the storage of energy in glycogen, Krebs cycle metabolism, and the ability to produce internal antioxidants.[16] That's a fancy way of saying they block the things that make us tired.

### Linoleic Acid

There are only two fats we need from our diets—linoleic acid (omega-6) and alpha-linolenic acid (omega-3). We need to get those two fats from foods for our bodies to function optimally. Together they regulate inflammation and the immune response. Fatigue is one of many issues that emerge when inflammation gets out of control. Many estimates list walnuts as the richest known source of linoleic acid. Other rich sources include sunflower seeds, pine nuts, and flaxseeds.

A recent study was done to compare the effects of essential fats on symptoms of fatigue as found in survivors of breast cancer. The researchers gave different groups of participants high doses of omega-6 fats or omega-3 fats. Prior to the study, they predicted that omega-3 fats would be more beneficial than omega-6. Yet the omega-6 fats from walnuts improved fatigue more than omega-3 fats. Those given omega-6 fats as found in walnuts were less tired and had lower levels of inflammatory markers like TNF-alpha.[17]

# Nutraceutical Solutions

## CORDYCEPS

*Cordyceps sinensis* is a type of fungus related to dietary mushrooms. It has been used as an energy tonic throughout Asia since the earliest recorded medical treatises.

Cordyceps is a premier example of an adaptogen. Adaptogens are plants and mushrooms containing phytonutrients that have been proven to increase resilience to a variety of stressors. A principle of Ayurvedic medicine is that there are three possible properties to a medicine. It can stimulate something, slow something, or help something regain balance. Drugs almost always stimulate or sedate something. They can do so in a broad sense in the form of stimulants that create alertness or sedatives that force sleep. They can also do that in a more specific manner, such as medications that stimulate or block a specific chemical pathway. Adaptogens are considered among the highest forms of treatment because they help your body respond to stress and fatigue, bringing your systems back to balance.

Cordyceps has been proven to improve energy by lowering thyroid antibodies, reducing inflammation, increasing antioxidant capacity, raising energy storage, and improving immune regulation. In one study, adults took capsules containing either cordyceps or a placebo for twelve weeks. Exercise performance increased by over 10 percent in those taking cordyceps, but not in those on placebos.[18]

## ELEUTHERO

*Eleutherococcus senticosus* (Siberian ginseng) is the root of an Asian plant with a long history of use as an energy tonic. It is known to act as an antioxidant, an immune tonic, and a blood sugar regulator.

In a recent placebo-controlled blinded human clinical trial, eighty-seven participants were selected to evaluate the effects of eleuthero on chronic stress. Compared with those on placebo, those receiving eleuthero showed improvements in symptoms of fatigue and depression.[19]

## L-CITRULLINE

L-citrulline (citrulline malate) is an amino acid that can improve exercise capacity. It is converted by the kidneys into L-arginine and nitric oxide.

In one study, women took L-citrulline or a placebo on two separate occasions. Those supplementing with L-citrulline showed a clear increase in strength without an increase in effort.[20]

---

*To learn more about how to use these and other nutraceutical ingredients, please visit the resources page at www.hormonehealing cookbook.com/resources.*

---

# CHAPTER 5

# Brain Fog

Brain fog is one of the newest symptoms of hormone imbalance, as well as one of the most distressing. I've surveyed my readers about their top symptoms for nearly two decades. In the past, some complained about forgetfulness or difficulty in concentrating. Sometimes they described episodes as senior moments. But none of these were common.

Starting in 2014, symptoms like those consolidated into one term—brain fog. Since then, it has rapidly become a top complaint among those with hormone imbalances. Brain fog is the inability to recall certain details—passwords, the name of an old friend, the reason you walked into another room. But it is more than that. Those who have it feel like they are quite literally stuck in fog. They can feel unclear about their direction, their purpose, and even their own feelings.

Many who experience it fear that it could be the first sign of a severe brain disease. Neurologists tell us that this is not the case. The early stages of conditions like Alzheimer's disease involve far more than simple forgetfulness—people lose good judgment and other critical thinking skills. But even if brain fog is not a harbinger of doom, it is unpleasant. So what causes it?

## Hidden Causes of Brain Fog

The more finely tuned a machine is, the more easily it can get out of balance. The human brain may be the most finely tuned machine in the known universe. Even if it is out of tune, it can manage our basic survival needs like respiration. But unless it is working at peak performance, we won't be able to experience higher feelings like happiness and vitality.

Nearly any medical problem can disrupt your brain. Sometimes simple causes

53

of brain fog can be found and fixed. Some of the more common ones include anemia, poorly regulated blood sugar, extra weight, and sleep apnea. If you suffer from brain fog, please do work with your doctor to see if any medical issues may be contributing to it. As we've seen with other symptoms, finding the cause is ideal, but help is possible even when a cause is not found. This is possible because it's exacerbated by a small number of mechanisms, no matter the cause—poor delivery of oxygen, inability to regulate glucose, unchecked inflammation, and free radical damage.

A poor delivery of oxygen can be caused by unremarkable factors like shallow breathing or early medical events like narrowed blood vessels. Poor glucose regulation is the central insult of diabetes, but it also happens from skipping meals and eating highly processed foods. Inflammation is normal, but autoimmune diseases or inactivity can cause the body to turn against itself. Free radicals are also unavoidable, but unmanageable quantities come from airborne pollutants and fried foods.

Even though these causes are numerous, the right foods can still make a big difference.

## Foods That Reverse Brain Fog

### BASIL

Basil is a delightful herb that can easily boost mental clarity. Fresh basil is great, but dried can work fine; you can even grow some on your windowsill. All these forms can improve mental function, and they do so in amounts that can easily be incorporated into your diet. In a recent controlled clinical study, adults who consumed basil were shown to have faster reaction times, lower error rates, and several other measurable improvements of mental function.[1]

I mentioned earlier that brain fog can go along with conditions like anxiety. Basil can help brain fog by itself, and it can ameliorate the anxiety that goes with it. One study proved that as anxiety levels improved, participants found it easier to concentrate.[2]

How does basil do this? Part of the effects come from a constituent called linalool. Preliminary studies have shown that linalool can boost cognitive function and improve mental clarity. Because linalool is found in all types of commercially available basil, you do not need to worry about the distinctions between, for example, Genovese basil, Thai basil, or holy basil.[3]

In the kitchen, basil can work well with a big range of dishes, both savory and sweet. I've got several for you in the recipe section that you won't find anywhere else! Even if you're not a fan of regular pesto, be sure to try my Avocado Spinach Pesto (page 218).

## BERRIES

If you forget the food lists, just remember—foods that stain heal your brain. Berries sure can stain! They stain because they are full of pigments like proanthocyanins, ellagitannins, stilbenoids, and more. These naturally occurring pigments break down free radicals and help our body deal with toxins. They keep our genes working right and help our immune system destroy cancer cells.

Berries also have the specific effect of improving word recall. If it seems the right words are always on the tip of your tongue, eat more berries. Studies have shown that adults with mild cognitive impairment given blueberry juice were able to retrieve words faster than otherwise.

In one such study, middle-aged adults had their mental function tested after a single dose of a berry smoothie. Those who drank it were able to do better on complex mental tasks. They also were able to concentrate for longer periods of time. The smoothie used in the study was nothing too exotic: 1½ ounces each of strawberries, blueberries, blackberries, and raspberries blended with 3 ounces of water.[4]

## LEAFY GREENS

The data is clear. Multiple high-quality studies show that those who eat dark leafy greens have healthier brains then those who do not. This relationship held true even after controlling for other factors that disrupt hormones including age, gender, education, exercise status, smoking, seafood intake, and alcohol usage.

Greens help because they offer essential micronutrients like K vitamins, folate, and carotenoids. There are many such nutrients we need that are just not found in high amounts in any other foods. Those who eat more greens are less apt to be low in them. Harmful gut bacteria make an enzyme called beta-glucuronidase, which causes hormone imbalances and poorer brain function. Those who eat more greens have lower levels of beta-glucuronidase.

Greens also have several novel phytonutrients that make the brain more resilient to daily stress. Some of the top such compounds found in leafy greens include:

- Alpha-tocopherol: an E vitamin that protects cells from fat-soluble free radicals.

- Lutein: a carotenoid found in many foods that improves the health of small blood vessels.

- Kaempferol: a polyphenol that lowers inflammation and helps the brain get rid of old cells.

- Nitrates: nitrogen-containing compounds that help oxygen reach the brain.

- Phylloquinone: one of the active K vitamins found in higher levels in centenarians (hundred-year-olds) with exceptional cognitive function.

In fact, those who averaged one additional serving per day had brains that functioned as if they were eleven years younger![5]

What are the best examples of leafy greens? My favorites include kale, collards, spinach, beet greens, watercress, romaine lettuce, Swiss chard, arugula, endive, cabbage, and turnip greens. While you can sneak spinach in almost any recipe with no one the wiser, the other greens do take some planning to integrate into a meal.

## ROSEMARY

Rosemary has been used in a variety of forms, including as a culinary spice, an ingredient in tea, and an essential oil. All these forms have been shown to have beneficial effects on cognitive function. The terpenes and terpenoids in rosemary can improve circulation and oxygen delivery to the brain.

Rosemary also works quickly. In fact, its benefits show up almost immediately. In one study, participants drank mineral water steeped with rosemary. A similar group drank plain mineral water. Both groups did cognitive tests. All participants were analyzed to see how much oxygen they had in their blood. Those ingesting rosemary did better on their mental tasks and enjoyed higher levels of blood oxygen.[6]

There are several kinds of rosemary commercially available. The type sold in spice jars and fresh in supermarkets is not the same as the one used as an ornamental plant. If you have some in your yard, it can still be used in the kitchen. You will likely need a third to a half as much as the rosemary found in supermarkets.

It's often used to season poultry and bean dishes. The easiest way to use it is to try my recipe for Rosemary Citrus Water (page 230). Use it as a beverage to help on days when you have lots of mental work ahead.

## TROUT

All evidence points to the fact that fish is a brain food. People who eat the most fish, whether saltwater or freshwater, have the healthiest brains. This is true for nearly any type of seafood—fish, shellfish, mollusks, or bivalves. Seafood in the diet reduces the risks for mild cognitive impairment, cognitive decline, and Alzheimer's disease.[7]

All kinds of seafood can be healthy, but some types have negative baggage to consider. These problems include excessive iodine, sustainability issues, or toxicants like BPA or mercury. Due to considerations like these, some of the best types to avoid include thresher shark, imported catfish, and Atlantic cod.

I chose freshwater trout as a top example because it has all the benefits and rarely any of the problems. It is easy to find, has a neutral taste, and is easy to prepare. Along with trout, I'll include recipes for other types of fish that are also good options.

The benefits of seafood show up without requiring you to eat massive amounts. Most studies suggest that two to three servings per week are all that it takes for full effects.

# Nutraceutical Solutions

## ASTRAGALUS

*Astragalus membranaceus* (Huangqi) is a root that has been used for thousands of years in China, both as a food and as a medicine. Because it is a food, it has an excellent safety profile. High-quality human studies have shown it can safely improve cognitive function, even after brain damage from strokes.[8]

## L-CARNITINE

L-carnitine is a naturally occurring amino acid that is essential for cellular energy production.

Clinical trials have shown that supplementation with L-carnitine can improve symptoms of mental fatigue in those with thyroid disease. In a representative study, sixty people with significant levels of fatigue were given L-carnitine or a placebo for twelve weeks. Those taking L-carnitine noticed clear improvements in fatigue severity, physical fatigue, and mental fatigue.[9]

## L-THEANINE

L-theanine is a naturally occurring nonprotein amino acid. It is found in foods such as mushrooms and tea—black, green, oolong, and white. In supplement form, theanine has been shown to improve cognitive function and decrease mental fatigue. In one study, thirty adults took theanine tablets or a placebo over a four-week period. Most subjects were female, and the average age was 48.3 years.

Depression, anxiety, sleep quality, and cognitive function scores all improved in those taking theanine. Verbal fluency also showed a marked improvement.[10]

---

*To learn more about how to use these and other nutraceutical ingredients, please visit the resources page at www.hormonehealing cookbook.com/resources.*

---

# CHAPTER 6

# Hot Flashes

Hot flashes are often the first symptom that make women suspect a hormone imbalance. It is one of the most obvious and disruptive symptoms imaginable. They can be caused by several things, but in almost all cases they are part of a woman's hormonal transition into menopause.

## Menopause

For a typical woman, menstrual cycles start to change in the mid-forties. First, they become erratic: periods might be skipped; others may be just weeks apart. This fluctuation in periods is correlated to a fluctuation in estrogen. The ovaries can vacillate between secreting too much and too little. This first change marks perimenopause. Finally, estrogen levels drop off and stay low. Then the woman's periods stop. During the twelve months after the cessation of periods, a woman is considered to be in menopause. The average woman becomes menopausal at fifty-one, but the range can be from the mid-thirties to age sixty. Once periods have been absent for a full year, the woman is considered postmenopausal and remains there for the rest of her life.

The hormone imbalance symptoms associated with menopause can happen during any part of the journey–perimenopause, menopause, and for some, even well into postmenopause. These symptoms include fatigue, poor sleep, weight gain, brain fog, dry skin, thinning hair, mood changes, a reduced sex drive, and vaginal dryness. Although those symptoms may appear in any combination, they are usually accompanied by hot flashes.

Hot flashes can be startling at first. They are usually described as distinct from any other symptom. Typically, they feel like quick bursts of heat, primarily on the skin, face, and neck. They last about thirty seconds to five minutes. Your skin may become visibly red, especially on the face. It is common to break out in a sweat and have a racing heart. After a hot flash stops, you may feel tired, irritable, and disoriented.

Most who get hot flashes have at least one per day. Some get only a few per week, and some are unlucky enough to get one every hour. For 10 to 15 percent of women, hot flashes are so bad they get in the way of life. Night sweats, hot flashes that happen at night, have the added frustration of disrupting sleep. We now know that as traumatic as hot flashes can be, they are also a warning sign. Large studies have shown that women who have the worst hot flashes are at higher risk for heart disease.[1]

## Andropause

Men undergo a similar hormonal disruption called andropause. A man's testosterone levels peak at adolescence and gradually decline for the rest of their life. But some men experience a dramatic drop-off in their mid-forties or mid-fifties. Andropause can also cause hot flashes. In one study, a third of men between the ages of fifty-five and seventy-five experienced hot flashes. Those who get them often have other symptoms of andropause such as decreased muscle strength or endurance, decreased enjoyment of life, sadness or grumpiness, and lack of energy.[2] The foods below that help menopause also help andropause because both are caused by rapid hormonal changes.

## How Foods Help

Foods that help your liver often help hot flashes. This is because hot flashes are caused by rapid imbalances in hormones, and a healthy liver can keep hormone levels steady. Foods can also improve hormone receptors. Hormones are like keys that fit specific locks. The body can adjust the number of receptors (the locks) and make them easier or harder to open. Phytonutrients can help all this exacting chemistry work more smoothly.

Specifically, in the case of hot flashes, isoflavones enable estrogen to be absorbed by some receptors while blocking it from others. In doing so, they can lower symptoms of too little estrogen like hot flashes, while protecting against the effects of too much, like breast cell proliferation.

Gene expression is another part of the hormone equation. Hormones activate or inhibit certain portions of genes. We know that when important reactions, like DNA methylation, slow down, estrogen cannot always be converted into safe by-products. Cruciferous vegetables improve gene expression so that estrogen can be safely eliminated.

# Foods for Brain Fog

The foods I've listed here will help ameliorate those hormonal symptoms. Please note that these foods largely work through different mechanisms. Don't feel like you need to eat each of these foods every day or at every meal. Think more about trying to include one or two of them on any given day. You'll likely see even greater benefits this way while not getting bored of repetition.

## CABBAGE AND OTHER CRUCIFEROUS VEGGIES

Cruciferous vegetables improve the intricate mechanisms your liver uses to keep estrogen levels stable. These include enzymes with esoteric names like cytochrome P450 1A1 and glutathione S-transferase.[3] These improvements are likely the reason cruciferous vegetables may protect against breast cancer.[4]

In a recent study, a group of breast cancer survivors were tracked to see if their diets related to menopausal symptoms. There was a direct relationship. The more cruciferous vegetables the participants ate, the milder their symptoms were.[5]

## CITRUS FRUITS

As mentioned above, hot flashes are worse in those prone to heart disease. It turns out that those with the worst hot flashes (over 10 per day) are likely to have inflexible blood vessels.[6] As the blood vessels get stiff, they are less able to expand and contract through a daily cycle. This stiffness drives up blood pressure and raises the risk for cardiovascular disease. It also seems to cause hot flashes.

In studies about food and menopausal symptoms, citrus fruits were shown to be the most effective of all food categories in reducing menopausal symptoms.[7]

## FIGS

Could figs be the forgotten fruit? Studies have shown that figs can significantly reduce the frequency and severity of hot flashes. One of the active compounds in figs is 7-methoxycoumarin (MC). Like estrogen, it can reduce hot flashes and heal the vaginal lining. Unlike estrogen, it is safe even in amounts thousands of times above what's found in food.[8]

Figs have other well-documented benefits to human health. Among fruits and vegetables, they are among the richest sources of minerals. They supply substantial amounts of calcium, iron, and potassium.

## SOY

Soy foods are widely used in the healthiest parts of the world but are less used in America. In recent years, soy has become a source of unwarranted controversy. Yet the studies are quite clear. Soy offers health benefits found in no other foods. Soy foods help prevent heart disease, breast cancer, and hip fractures.[9] They also improve menopausal symptoms. Soy does not disrupt thyroid function or cause cancer. Soy does not contain estrogen. Its isoflavonoids can both boost the good effects of estrogen and block its bad effects—helping both versions of a hormone imbalance.

As we discussed earlier, hormones like estrogen work once they connect to receptors on cells. There are multiple types of estrogen receptors. One type, called alpha receptors, is found in cells of the skin, brain, and bones. The other type, called beta receptors, is found in breast cells and those of the endometrium. Estrogen is "good" when it activates alpha receptors. It makes for healthier skin, stronger bones, better cognitive function, and fewer hot flashes. It is "bad" when it activates beta receptors. Then it is a culprit behind breast cancer and endometrial hyperplasia.

Soy gives you the best of both worlds. It stimulates alpha receptors while blocking the beta receptors. That is why it can do things that seem contradictory, like prevent breast cancer and improve hot flashes. Soy even helps those who have had hormonally sensitive breast cancer. Those who eat more soy have better odds of avoiding recurrence and of surviving.[10]

Many women see clear reductions in hot flashes with even modest amounts of soy foods. For the average woman, it takes one to two servings most days per week. Each day, you can incorporate one or two of the following:

- Soy milk in place of dairy milk
- Soy yogurt with breakfast
- Tofu in place of animal protein
- Soy sauce as a condiment
- Edamame as a snack
- Miso soup with a meal

## TURMERIC

Turmeric has become known as a go-to food for lowering inflammation. It has a constituent called curcumin that does many of the useful things anti-inflammatory medications can do, with fewer side effects.[11] Many do not know that it has also been shown to reduce hot flashes.

In a blind randomized study, ninety-three women received a turmeric extract or a placebo for eight weeks. Within four weeks, those taking turmeric saw their hot flashes reduced by half. Within four more weeks, the women taking turmeric had over a fourfold reduction in their number of hot flashes. The amount of turmeric extract used was just 1 gram daily. This amount is easy to get from food alone.[12]

# Nutraceutical Solutions

## HUMULUS

The plant *Humulus lupulus,* the common hop or hops, is a rich source of phytonutrients, especially varieties of flavones and chalcones. One chalcone, called 8-prenylnaringenin, has been shown to reduce hot flashes and improve other menopausal symptoms. In a double-blind, placebo-controlled study, sixty-seven women were given capsules containing either *Humulus lupulus* or a placebo for twelve weeks and monitored for menopausal symptoms. Compared with the placebo, those using *H. lupulus* enjoyed significant reductions in hot flashes and other menopausal symptoms.[13]

## S-EQUOL

Soy foods greatly reduce menopausal symptoms in some women, but not all. It turns out those who benefit are those whose gut flora can convert soy compounds into S-equol. Since many cannot do so, S-equol can be used directly. Even though it is not a hormone, S-equol may be more effective than hormone replacement therapy for the alleviation of hot flashes.[14]

---

*To learn more about how to use these and other nutraceutical ingredients, please visit the resources page at www.hormonehealing cookbook.com/resources.*

---

# CHAPTER 7

# Insomnia

More people are realizing how important sleep is to their overall health, but many still don't realize how poor sleep can worsen almost any symptom imaginable.

Nearly every known function of the body works on a circadian rhythm. The daily cycle is one of getting things done. It is a time of activity, higher metabolism, movement, and mental activity. The nightly cycle is one of repair, maintenance, and preparation for the next day.

Of the hormones we've introduced, melatonin and cortisol do the most to regulate this rhythm. Our hypothalamus stimulates the adrenal glands to release a burst of cortisol in the morning called the cortisol awakening response. Think of it like a built-in coffeepot with an automatic timer. The cortisol surge comes on about an hour before waking and gradually tapers off throughout the day.

In the late afternoon, cortisol levels drop off abruptly. The rapid decline of cortisol triggers the pineal gland to release melatonin. You could imagine cortisol and melatonin sitting on opposite sides of a seesaw. When one goes up, the other goes down. Melatonin peaks just before bedtime and makes us sleepy. The pineal gland keeps making a little bit throughout the night to keep us asleep. The next morning, the cortisol awakening response kicks in and shuts off melatonin until the next night.

Every part of the body is a cluster of distinct cells—brain cells, muscle cells, skin cells, and so on. Some cells live for just a few minutes, some a few years. All of them must be replaced regularly. Deep sleep is essential for the breakdown of old cells and the growth of new ones. Sleep is also essential for the proper storage of food as fuel. With sleep, calories can be stored in the liver and muscles in ways that allow it to be easily retrieved. With too little sleep, the same calories can be stored only as visceral fat. This type of stored fuel is harder to get to and a problematic source of inflammation.

Could better sleep help you? To answer that, think about how you feel while on vacation. Do you feel happier and more alert? Does life seem to flow better? It has been argued that most of the boost we get from vacations comes from extra sleep. Wouldn't it be great to have some of that every day?

# Types and Symptoms of Insomnia

There are lots of ways sleep can go wrong. I'll share some of the different types here, in case any of these sleep issues seem familiar to you. Hopefully, you can start to improve your sleep quality with the food solutions offered in this book.

Chronic insomnia is defined by the inability to sleep well for three or more days per week for a month or longer. Any less than that is intermittent insomnia. Chronic insomnia can be called primary when it happens by itself, or secondary when it is caused by other medical issues.

Acute insomnia encompasses issues like jet lag, sleeping in a new place, or poor sleep from sudden grief. One can have an issue with either falling asleep (sleep onset), staying asleep (sleep maintenance), or both. Those who cannot fall asleep without sleep aids are considered to have sleep onset issues.

Besides problems with being able to sleep, some suffer from unrefreshing sleep. Some people can sleep when they want, but don't feel like they had enough even when it seems they did. Because sleep affects the entire body's ability to heal, poor sleep can cause nearly any symptom. Sleep disturbances can cause daytime sleepiness, irritability, and difficulty in concentrating. Other symptoms of poor sleep are often not thought of as such. Top symptoms can include easy weight gain, susceptibility to injury, headaches, and poor digestion.

# Finding the Cause

In recent years we've learned that poor sleep is more than a nuisance. It raises the risk for heart disease, diabetes, and some cancers, and shortens the lifespan.[1]

For many, poor sleep is the first sign of menopause or andropause. If sleep has been a severe problem throughout all your life, consider professional help. Talk to your doctor about possible medical issues and see if you should have a referral to a sleep specialist. Sleep studies are much less invasive than in the past and can often be done at home. Many people have sleep apnea or other treatable issues they would never otherwise have been aware of.

You may be able to identify milder sleep problems on your own. No matter what, recipes to improve sleep can be helpful. Here are several factors that can lead to poor sleep and other symptoms of a hormone imbalance.

## CAFFEINE AND INSOMNIA

If your sleep quality is poor, caffeine could be a culprit. Even if you have only one cup of coffee per day, it can be enough to disrupt your sleep. For some people, even small amounts of caffeine can lead to difficulty falling asleep, difficulty staying asleep, poor sleep quality, and daytime sleepiness.[2] Caffeine can affect us differently as we age. There are those who did fine with it when they were younger but find it problematic as they grow older. When testing this in yourself, be sure to avoid all sources so you can know for sure. Look for caffeine in coffee, tea, chocolate, medications, supplements, and endurance foods like gels. Skip it for three weeks and see if things change. If not, you can always add it back to your diet.

If you find that caffeine does affect your sleep, that doesn't mean you can never have it again. Many find it works better to skip caffeine one or two days per week than it does to have a smaller amount daily.

## LACK OF EXERCISE

Do you know how much harder kids sleep when they're well played out? Well, it is the same for adults! Physical movement is necessary for the body's circadian changes that help us fall asleep. The most effective starting place can be a twenty-minute walk after dinner. Doing this helps to lower cortisol and kick in the body's own production of melatonin, which leads to sleep.

## PRIORITIZE SLEEP

How many hours of sleep do you get when you don't have to wake early? If you normally get less than this, you may benefit by allocating more time for sleep. Try to avoid sleeping later some days than others. Your body quickly anchors the later sleep time and considers it to be normal. When you wake up earlier, it can feel like you have jet lag. You are forcing your body to get up before it is ready. People have long tried to find ways to hack sleep so that they can function on less sleep, but the consensus among sleep researchers is that all these attempts do is make people used to performing badly.

## SLEEP HYGIENE

It seems that many of our modern comforts were designed to keep us from sleeping! Some of the most helpful sleep hygiene tips start in the morning.

Each morning, spend half an hour or more outdoors in the sun—ideally within the first hour of waking. Morning sun resets the circadian rhythm inside your body that triggers sleep fourteen to sixteen hours later. At night, give yourself a good hour before bed to wind down. Put away the electronics, dim the lights, and if possible, lower your home's temperature by 5 or more degrees Fahrenheit. Make your room as dark as possible. If that is difficult, consider an eye mask. If sounds bother you, consider masking them with white noise or wearing earplugs. Some earplugs are specially made for sleep and won't fall out when you roll on your side.

# Foods to Improve Sleep

We have good evidence that the right foods can improve sleep. In the remainder of the chapter, I'll talk about how specific foods and particular nutrients from food can help you fall asleep quickly and have more refreshing sleep.

## BLACK RICE

Black rice made this list for three reasons. First, healthy carbs at night can improve sleep. Second, diets higher in rice specifically are shown to improve sleep quality. In one study, jasmine rice given an hour before bedtime significantly decreased the time required for sleep onset.[3] Third, black rice is a rich source of polyphenols and plant melatonin—both of which can improve sleep.

### Why Carbs Help

Regular sleep depends upon hormones like serotonin and melatonin. Diets that are too low in carbohydrates can lower both of those sleep hormones and create an imbalance.

In a study, a group of women was put on a low-carbohydrate diet to see how it might alter their sleep stages. Their calorie intake was controlled so that they were not consuming more or fewer calories than typical. Within two days, their REM sleep was reduced by 19 percent.[4]

Low-carb diets are usually higher in fat. Dietary fat causes the release of a hormone called cholecystokinin (CCK), which makes us feel full and sleepy. However, when CCK is too high, it impairs sleep quality.[5] Striking the right balance is important.

### Unique Compounds in Black Rice

Polyphenols are plant pigments and are found in several colorful plant foods such as black rice, blueberries, artichokes, and flaxseeds.[6] In an Italian study, those who ate the most polyphenols were shown to have the best quality of sleep.[7] Research has shown that polyphenols may also improve brain function in several ways. They have been shown to lower the risks for conditions including:

- Insomnia
- Depression
- Dementia
- Alzheimer's disease

Black rice is one of the densest plant sources of melatonin and polyphenols.[8]

## CHERRIES

There is good evidence attesting to the role of cherries as a sleep aid. In one study, people over fifty with insomnia were given cherry juice or a placebo. Those receiving cherry juice showed dramatic increases in melatonin. They slept longer and had better-quality sleep. It seems that cherries helped the participants produce melatonin, because the elevation was greater than could be explained by the cherries alone.[9]

In those over sixty-five, insomnia is associated with an increased risk for falls. These are a big deal. Falling is the most common cause of hip fractures, and those who break their hip have a 50 percent risk of mortality in the following year. When seniors are given drugs to help them sleep, their risk for falls goes up over fourfold.[10] Cherries were able to effectively treat insomnia in older adults without increasing their risk for falls.[11]

## KIWI

Kiwifruit is rich in sleep-improving compounds, including antioxidants and melatonin. Since rumors abounded about the ability of kiwis to improve sleep, a group of scientists decided to test them out. They had a group of adults eat two kiwis before bed each night for four weeks. The duration and the quality of their sleep were tracked via surveys and wearable devices. The kiwis caused them to fall asleep 35 percent faster. They also woke up less often after going to sleep and saw an improvement of over 40 percent in their sleep quality index scores.[12]

## POULTRY

Perhaps you've heard that turkey has tryptophan and that's why we get tired after eating on Thanksgiving. This piece of holiday lore contains a kernel of truth as well as several misunderstandings.

The main regulator of sleep is the hormone melatonin. Your body makes it from serotonin, which is in turn made from tryptophan. Tryptophan is an essential amino acid found in a variety of foods. Other amino acids compete with tryptophan for passage across the blood-brain barrier. Foods that have the most dramatic effect on serotonin production

are those with the most tryptophan relative to their other amino acids.

Lean poultry is the star of the show when it comes to dietary sources. When ranking sources of tryptophan by calorie, various forms of poultry take seven of the top ten spots. Chicken is higher in tryptophan than turkey, but turkey has fewer competing amino acids. Insulin pulls those competing amino acids out of the bloodstream. When the level of other amino acids is lower, tryptophan can make serotonin. The fatigue after Thanksgiving has more to do with overeating than it does with turkey. Otherwise, chicken would make us sleepier than turkey.[13] As we age, our bodies can have a harder time producing serotonin and responding to it. Clinical trials have shown that improving tryptophan in the diet can help. In one study, raising dietary tryptophan improved sleep onset and sleep time, and reduced symptoms of anxiety.[14] In such studies, tryptophan-rich foods are used throughout the day, not just at bedtime.

## Top Food Sources of Tryptophan
(per 200-calorie serving sizes)[15]

| | |
|---|---|
| Lean chicken breast | 515 mg |
| Fat-free broiled turkey patties | 478 mg |
| Ground turkey | 477 mg |
| Turkey drumstick | 462 mg |
| Roasted turkey, light meat | 437 mg |

## PISTACHIOS

Like people, plants respond to cycles of day and night. They make melatonin to help control these cycles, and some contain enough melatonin to help us sleep when we eat them.

The melatonin found in plants can be absorbed, just as it can from supplements. Researchers have tracked participants' levels of melatonin before and after they consume melatonin-rich plants. Not only do we absorb melatonin from food, but it causes us to make more of our own. Gram per gram, pistachios are far higher in melatonin than any other food, fungi, spice, or medicinal herb. Assays have shown that pistachios can have 230 micrograms of melatonin per gram of dry weight. This amount equates to over 6,000 micrograms of melatonin per a 1-ounce serving.[16]

# Nutraceutical Solutions

By far the most studied and talked about nutraceutical is melatonin. There is good evidence that it can be safely used to adjust sleep timing and speed sleep onset. However, the doses of melatonin in supplements are not based on evidence.

If a dose of melatonin is too low or too high, it does not work as well. Excessive doses also cause disturbed dreams and daytime fatigue. How much is too high? Most studies suggest 50 to 100 micrograms as an optimal dose for adults. Most products contain twenty to a hundred times that amount![17]

The best versions of melatonin are in the optimal dosage range and are immediately absorbed. Many studies have shown that when taken in doses of 100 to 200 micrograms, melatonin can be a safe way for adults to correct occasional insomnia and regain a normal sleep schedule. The problem is that nearly all products contain much higher doses, usually ten to a hundred times higher. Such megadose melatonin tends to be less effective because the body creates a resistance against the high dose. The other problem with a megadose of melatonin is that it cannot be cleared from the body before morning, leading to daytime grogginess. You can learn more about an effective version of melatonin called Thyrotonin at www.hormone healingcookbook.com/resources.

# PART 3

# Meal Plans & Recipes

# CHAPTER 8

# Meal Plans & Shopping Lists

If you wish to eat healthily and keep your hormones balanced, you can use all of the recipes in this book. You are welcome to pick and choose as you see fit. If you have one symptom that you'd like to focus on, I've included five 14-Day Menu Plans that will help. They are built around the most helpful ingredients for the symptom of your choice. Before you get started, here are some insights to help you better make use of the plans.

Each meal plan has shopping lists for week 1 and week 2. They are made assuming you are cooking all meals for four adults. If you are cooking for just one or two, please adjust accordingly. Each shopping list will include perishables and pantry items. In most cases you'll need to purchase the perishables, but you'll probably have most of the pantry items already in stock. Just double-check to be sure. If you'd like PDF versions of the shopping lists that you can print, you can find them at: www .hormonehealingcookbook.com/resources.

In my home, we have three meals a day, and each consists of three or more different dishes—usually a main dish and two sides. I think of the parts of a meal as veggies, carbs, and protein. Fat is important as well, but it usually works its way in through secondary ingredients like cooking oil or the fat naturally found in foods. Altogether we're talking about nine dishes each day. I'd guess you don't have time to cook nine dishes. I sure don't, so I've made it easier for you.

Each of the 14 days will have one to two distinct recipes. The rest of your meals can come from planned leftovers, precooked staples, and easy standby dishes. Planned leftovers are just that. The most common example will be lunch from dinner's leftovers.

Most days I'll suggest making more dinner than you need so that you will intentionally have leftovers for tomorrow's lunch. An easy habit is to dish up and refrigerate your food container for tomorrow at the same time you dish up plates for dinner. It also helps with portion control. I've put that strategy to work for you in the meal plans. You'll find that many meals suggest cooking in a larger quantity to use for the following day.

You may also note that most weekday breakfasts and lunches will require little time. They are either recipes that take just a few minutes or include leftovers from yesterday's dinner. Some of the weekend breakfast and lunch dishes are more involved, since people typically have more time. The meal plans suggest Saturday as the main day for shopping and food preparation. Check your shopping list and get everything you need for the coming week. Experiment with prepping your veggies before you put them away. It saves so much time during the week. Peel and dice root veggies and refrigerate. Dice onions, package, and freeze. Wash greens and place in a bag with cloth or paper towels and refrigerate.

Remember, any of these recipes can be used on the Maintenance Plan on any of my other programs: the Adrenal Reset Diet, the Metabolism Reset Diet, and the Thyroid Reset Diet. In each recipe, I've included modifications, if needed, for the Reset phases of these diet plans. I've also included gluten-free and vegan options for each recipe.

# After the 14 Days

Three possible scenarios may emerge by the end of the 14 days, each with different solutions.

*Scenario 1. Your symptom did improve, but you have another you'd like help with.* This will likely be the case for most people. Has the first symptom improved as much as you'd like? If so, move on to the 14-Day Menu Plan that corresponds to your next highest priority symptom. If not, consider repeating your last 14-Day Menu Plan and refer to scenario 2.

*Scenario 2. Your symptom has not been resolved.* My first suggestion would be to repeat the 14-Day Menu Plan. Some symptoms that respond well to dietary change may require two to three months to fully improve. You might also reread the chapter about that symptom to see if there are any other helpful steps you could also try or other causes that you might investigate.

*Scenario 3. Your symptom has been resolved, and you have no other symptoms.* That's awesome! You're welcome to pick and choose among all the recipes as you see fit. If you like the simplicity of the planned menus and shopping lists, you can also follow any of the 14-Day Menu Plans.

# 14 Days of Weight Loss

*Featured Foods: Cayenne, Ginger, Lentils, Onions*

## WEEK 1

| | BREAKFAST | LUNCH | DINNER |
|---|---|---|---|
| SUNDAY | Cayenne Scrambled Eggs (page 125) | Healthy Niçoise Salad (page 209) | Cactus Chili (page 202), Homemade Pickled Ginger (page 227) |
| MONDAY | Shake Template (page 107) | Leftovers from Sunday | Onion Skin Rice (page 163), Baked Chicken (page 139), Steamed Broccoli (page 192) |
| TUESDAY | Beet Green Smoothie (page 109) | Leftovers from Monday | Cucumber Salad with Ginger Dressing (page 175), Onion Skin Rice (page 163), Baked Chicken (page 139) |
| WEDNESDAY | Basic Oatmeal (page 111) | Leftovers from Tuesday | Healthy Niçoise Salad (page 209) |
| THURSDAY | Shake Template (page 107) | Leftovers from Wednesday | Seasoned Lentils (page 158), Roasted Root Veggies (page 190) |
| FRIDAY | Carob Fig Balls (page 124) | Leftovers from Thursday | Lentil Avocado Smash (page 156), Roasted Root Veggies (page 190) |
| SATURDAY | Shake Template (page 107) | Sesame Orange Chicken (page 134) | Dr. C's Potato Salad (page 165), Shredded Chicken (page 152) |

## WEEK 2

| | BREAKFAST | LUNCH | DINNER |
|---|---|---|---|
| SUNDAY | Spiced Banana Bread (page 126) | Ginger Garlic Stir-Fry (page 204) | Garlic Mashed Potatoes (page 167), Shredded Chicken (page 152), Steamed Broccoli (page 192) |
| MONDAY | Shake Template (page 107) | Leftovers from Sunday | Gingered Collards (page 182), Poached Trout (page 147), brown rice |
| TUESDAY | Turmeric Banana Shake (page 106) | Leftovers from Monday | Lean French Onion Soup (page 185), Artisan Bread (page 170), Poached Trout (page 147) |
| WEDNESDAY | Basic Oatmeal (page 111) | Leftovers from Tuesday | Ginger Garlic Stir-Fry (page 204) |
| THURSDAY | Apple Almond Shake (page 108) | Leftovers from Wednesday | Shrimp and Spicy Rice Noodles (page 213) |
| FRIDAY | Shake Template (page 107) | Leftovers from Thursday | Caramelized Onion Pudding (page 159), Shredded Chicken (page 152) |
| SATURDAY | Basic Oatmeal (page 111) | Minestrone Meatloaf (page 211) | Lentil Veggie Soup (page 210) |

# Week 1 Shopping List (4 Adults)

## PANTRY STAPLES

### Spices

Bay leaves

Black pepper

Cayenne pepper

Chili powder

Cumin, ground

Kosher salt

Paprika

Red pepper flakes

Turmeric powder

Vanilla extract

### Condiments

Apple cider vinegar

Dijon mustard

Honey

Neutral cooking oil
(avocado, canola,
grapeseed)

Olive oil

Rice vinegar

Tamari soy sauce

### Others

Arrowroot/cornstarch

Basmati rice

Brown rice

Carob powder

Flax milk, unsweetened

Nutritional yeast
(folic-acid-free)

Rolled oats

Stevia

Sucanat

White sesame seeds

## NONPERISHABLES

1 pound whole almonds

1 (3.5-ounce) jar capers

1 (8-ounce) pack dried figs

1 (10-ounce) jar
kalamata olives

1 (14.5-ounce) can
kidney beans

1 pound dried lentils

1 (19-ounce) jar nopalitos

1 (12-ounce) jar pickle relish

Protein powder:
Top picks include pea
or soy protein with at
least 22 grams of protein
per serving.

1 (14.5-ounce) can
diced tomatoes

1 (4-ounce) can tomato paste

2 (14.5-ounce) cans
tomato sauce

4 (5-ounce) cans
skipjack tuna

1 (32-ounce) carton
vegetable broth

## PERISHABLES

### Produce

2 medium avocados

1 pound baby carrots

2 bananas

2 bunches beets with greens

3 heads broccoli

1 bunch cilantro

1 medium cucumber

1 pint cherry tomatoes

1 package fresh dill, at least ½ ounce

4 servings fresh or frozen fruit for shakes (bananas, berries, or others)

2 bulbs garlic

¼ pound gingerroot

1 pound green beans

4 lemons

1 head butter lettuce

2 heads romaine lettuce

1 lime

1 (8-ounce) container white button mushrooms

4 medium onions

3 navel oranges

1 bunch fresh oregano

2 pounds Yukon Gold potatoes

2 pounds russet potatoes

1 medium red onion

1 red bell pepper

4 pounds root vegetables of choice (potatoes, sweet potatoes, beets, turnip, etc.)

1 bunch scallions

3 medium shallots

10 ounces spinach leaves

1 bunch fresh tarragon

1 bunch fresh thyme

1 medium tomato

1 (10- to 16-ounce) pack frozen mango

### Protein and Dairy

1 pound lean (90-97%) ground beef

9 pounds chicken breast

3 dozen eggs

# Daily Notes for Week 1

### SUNDAY

Big day in the kitchen today. If your schedule is tight, you can make enough food at lunch for dinner and leftovers (I suggest the Cactus Chili). Consider making the Baked Chicken today and refrigerating.

### THURSDAY

Carob Fig Balls are scheduled for tomorrow's breakfast. They don't take long—you might want to make them tonight and have them ready to go in the refrigerator for morning.

### SATURDAY

Tonight and tomorrow you will use Shredded Chicken. Find some time to make a large batch. I'd also suggest cooking up tomorrow's Spiced Banana Bread in advance if you can.

# Week 2 Shopping List (4 Adults)

## PANTRY STAPLES

### Spices

Bay leaves

Black pepper

Cayenne pepper

Garlic powder

Kosher salt

Paprika

Turmeric powder

Vanilla extract

### Condiments

Apple cider vinegar

Neutral cooking oil
(avocado, canola,
grapeseed)

Olive oil

Tamari soy sauce

Toasted sesame oil

### Others

All-purpose flour
(unbleached/unenriched)

Arrowroot/cornstarch

Baking powder
(aluminum-free)

Baking soda

Bread flour

Brown rice

Flax milk,
unsweetened

Rolled oats

Stevia

Sucanat

White sesame seeds

White wine

Whole wheat flour

## NONPERISHABLES

1 (8-ounce) jar
unsweetened applesauce

3 (32-ounce) cartons
beef broth

1 (14.5-ounce) can
cannellini beans

1 pound whole grain pasta

Peanut butter, crunchy

Protein powder:
Top picks include pea
or soy protein with at
least 22 grams of protein
per serving.

1 (12-ounce) package
rice noodles

1 (14.5-ounce) can diced
tomatoes

1 (4-ounce) can tomato paste

1 (32-ounce) carton
vegetable broth

## PERISHABLES

### Produce

1 Granny Smith apple

2 pounds carrots

4 bananas

5 heads broccoli

1 pint cherry tomatoes

1 bunch chives

1 bunch collard greens

1 package frozen edamame
(without pods)

4 servings fresh or frozen fruit for shakes (bananas, berries, or others)

3 bulbs garlic

¼ pound gingerroot

2 fresh jalapeño peppers

1 lemon

16 ounces white button mushrooms

4 medium onions

2 medium sweet onions

1 bunch fresh oregano

1 red bell pepper

1 pound red potatoes

3 pounds Yukon Gold potatoes

10 ounces spinach leaves

1 bunch fresh thyme

2 pounds zucchini

## Protein and Dairy

4 pounds chicken breast

1 dozen eggs

4 pounds trout fillets

1 pound lean (90-97%) ground turkey

1 pound fresh or frozen shrimp, large (21-29 per pound)

# Daily Notes for Week 2

## SUNDAY

Feel free to exchange dinner and lunch recipes. If you have leftovers, they can also be used for either meal.

## MONDAY

Tonight's protein is Poached Trout. You can make up extra for tomorrow night as well. Just be sure to slightly undercook that batch.

If you want to try tomorrow's Spiced Banana Bread, you're welcome to prepare the batter or bake it as well. We'll have some bread tomorrow. You can make it then or start it now and give it an extra day to ferment.

## WEDNESDAY

Pretty easy day. You'll need Shredded Chicken tomorrow and the next day. You can do it today or tomorrow.

## SATURDAY

You're finished! Time to make your next plans. Another 14-Day Menu Plan? Repeat some favorites? Try recipes outside of a plan?

# 14-Day Menu Plan for Energy

*Featured Foods: Almonds, Beets, Garlic, Oats, Walnuts*

## WEEK 1

| | BREAKFAST | LUNCH | DINNER |
|---|---|---|---|
| SUNDAY | Savory Spicy Granola (page 119) | Almond Chicken Sauté (page 138) | Curried Almond Squash Soup (page 179), Shredded Chicken (page 152), brown rice |
| MONDAY | Shake Template (page 107) | Leftovers from Sunday | Minestrone Meatloaf (page 211) |
| TUESDAY | Beet Green Smoothie (page 109) | Leftovers from Monday | Baked Chicken (page 139) with Garlic Lemon Sauce (page 222), brown rice |
| WEDNESDAY | Basic Oatmeal (page 111) | Leftovers from Tuesday | Garlic Mashed Potatoes (page 167), Poached Trout (page 147), Steamed Broccoli (page 192) |
| THURSDAY | Shake Template (page 107) | Leftovers from Wednesday | Roasted Garlic Spread (page 219) on Artisan Bread (page 170), Poached Trout (page 147), spinach leaves with Sesame Soy Dressing (page 223) |
| FRIDAY | Two-Ingredient Granola (page 118), Shake Template (page 107) | Leftovers from Thursday | Classic Walnut Pesto (page 220) on Artisan Bread (page 170), Baked Chicken (page 139) |
| SATURDAY | Peach Walnut Cobbler (page 123), Shake Template (page 107) | Beet Slaw (page 193), Artisan Bread (page 170), Baked Tofu (page 137) | Steel Cut Oat Risotto (page 162), Baked Chicken (page 139), Steamed Broccoli (page 192) |

## WEEK 2

| | BREAKFAST | LUNCH | DINNER |
|---|---|---|---|
| SUNDAY | Shake Template (page 107) | Minestrone Meatloaf (page 211) | Rosemary Citrus Chicken (page 151), Roasted Root Veggies (with beets) (page 190) |
| MONDAY | Shake Template (page 107) | Leftovers from Sunday | Garlic Mashed Potatoes (page 167), Baked Chicken (page 139), Daily Salad (page 178) |
| TUESDAY | Savory Spicy Granola (page 119), Shake Template (page 107) | Leftovers from Monday | Beet Slaw (page 193), Baked Tofu (page 137), Peach Walnut Cobbler (page 123) |
| WEDNESDAY | Basic Oatmeal (page 111) | Leftovers from Tuesday | Green Chili with Chicken (page 205) |
| THURSDAY | Apple Almond Shake (page 108) | Leftovers from Wednesday | Shredded Chicken (page 152), Classic Walnut Pesto (page 220) served over pasta, Daily Salad (page 178) |
| FRIDAY | Shake Template (page 107) | Leftovers from Thursday | Shredded Chicken (page 152), Roasted Garlic Spread (page 219) served over Artisan Bread (page 170), Steamed Broccoli (page 192) |
| SATURDAY | Beet Cookies (page 160), Shake Template (page 107) | Minestrone Meatloaf (page 211) | Almond Chicken Sauté (page 138) |

# Week 1 Shopping List (4 Adults)

## PANTRY STAPLES

### Spices

Bay leaves

Black pepper

Cayenne pepper

Curry powder

Garlic powder

Kosher salt

Paprika, smoked

Red pepper flakes

Thyme, dried

White pepper

### Condiments

Honey

Neutral cooking oil
(avocado, canola,
grapeseed)

Olive oil

Rice vinegar

Tamari soy sauce

Toasted sesame seed oil

### Others

Arrowroot/cornstarch

Basmati rice

Bread flour

Brown rice

Flax milk, unsweetened

Nutritional yeast
(folic-acid-free)

Rolled oats

Stevia

Sucanat

Whole wheat flour

## NONPERISHABLES

1 pound whole almonds

1 (14.5-ounce) can
cannellini beans

1 (8-ounce) jar maple syrup

1 pound whole grain pasta

Protein powder:
Top picks include pea or
soy protein with at least
22 grams of protein per
serving.

1 (14.5-ounce) can diced
tomatoes

1 (14.5-ounce) can tomato
paste

1 (32-ounce) carton
vegetable broth

1 (8-ounce) package
walnuts

## PERISHABLES

### Produce

8 ounces fresh basil

1 bunch beets with greens

4 heads broccoli

1 bunch fresh chives

1 bunch cilantro

4 servings fresh or frozen fruit for shakes (bananas, berries, or others)

2 bulbs garlic

¼ pound gingerroot

3 lemons

2 limes

1 (10- to 16-ounce) pack frozen mango

1 (8-ounce) pack mushrooms

2 medium onions

2 medium sweet onions

1 bunch fresh oregano

3 pounds peaches

1 pound frozen peas

2 pounds Yukon Gold potatoes

4 pounds root vegetables of choice (potatoes, sweet potatoes, beets, turnips, etc.)

1 bunch scallions

10 ounces spinach leaves

1 kabocha squash

1 pound zucchini

### Protein and Dairy

9 pounds chicken breast

1 dozen eggs

1 (1-pound) package frozen peas

2 (15-ounce) blocks extra-firm tofu

1 pound trout fillets

1 pound lean (90–97%) ground turkey

# Daily Notes for Week 1

## SUNDAY

When you cook brown rice tonight, make some extra and refrigerate it for Tuesday's dinner.

## WEDNESDAY

Tonight's protein is Poached Trout. You can make up extra for tomorrow night as well; just be sure to slightly undercook that batch.

## THURSDAY

Are your mornings rushed? If so, make up tomorrow morning's Two-Ingredient Granola in advance. You can also make a double batch of Baked Chicken for the next two days.

## SATURDAY

Shopping day! Check your shopping list.

# Week 2 Shopping List (4 Adults)

## PANTRY STAPLES

### Spices

Bay leaves

Black pepper

Cinnamon, ground

Cumin, ground

Garlic salt

Kosher salt

Oregano, dried

Thyme, dried

Vanilla extract

White pepper

### Condiments

Apple cider vinegar

Dijon mustard

Neutral cooking oil
   (avocado, canola,
   grapeseed)

Olive oil

Tamari soy sauce

Toasted sesame oil

### Others

All-purpose flour
   (unbleached/unenriched)

Arrowroot/cornstarch

Baking powder
   (aluminum-free)

Baking soda

Bread flour

Brown rice

Flax milk, unsweetened

Maple syrup

Rolled oats

Stevia

Sucanat

Tapioca flour

Whole wheat flour

## NONPERISHABLES

1 pound whole almonds

1 jar almond butter

2 (32-ounce) cartons
   chicken broth

3 (14.5-ounce) cans
   cannellini beans

1 pound whole grain pasta

Protein powder: Top picks
   include pea or soy
   protein with at least
   22 grams of protein per
   serving.

1 (8-ounce or larger)
   container green
   chili salsa

1 (14.5-ounce) can diced
   tomatoes

1 (4-ounce) can tomato paste

1 (32-ounce) carton
   vegetable broth

1 (8-ounce) package
   walnuts

## PERISHABLES

### Produce

1 Granny Smith apple

8 ounces fresh basil

1 bunch beets

2 heads broccoli

1 pound carrots

2 cucumbers

4 servings fresh or frozen fruit for shakes (bananas, berries, or others)

4 bulbs garlic

¼ pound gingerroot

2 medium jicamas

1 pound leeks

3 lemons

16 ounces white button mushrooms

4 medium onions

2 medium sweet onions

1 bunch fresh oregano

1 bunch fresh parsley

3 pounds peaches

1 pound frozen peas

1 pound red potatoes

3 pounds Yukon Gold potatoes

4 pounds root vegetables of choice (potatoes, sweet potatoes, beets, turnips, etc.)

1 bunch fresh rosemary

1 bunch radishes

1 bunch scallions

10 ounces spinach leaves

2 pounds zucchini

### Protein and Dairy

9 pounds chicken breast

1 dozen eggs

2 (15-ounce) blocks extra-firm tofu

2 pounds lean (90-97%) ground turkey

# Daily Notes for Week 2

## SUNDAY

Baked Chicken for tonight and tomorrow—be sure to make a double batch.

## TUESDAY

Baked Tofu for tonight and tomorrow—be sure to prepare a double batch.

## THURSDAY

Shredded Chicken for tonight and tomorrow—be sure to make a double batch.

## SATURDAY

You're finished! Time to make your next plans. Another 14-Day Menu Plan? Repeat some favorites? Try recipes outside of a plan?

# 14-Day Menu Plan for Mental Clarity

*Featured Foods: Basil, Berries, Greens, Rosemary, Trout*

**WEEK 1**

| | BREAKFAST | LUNCH | DINNER |
|---|---|---|---|
| SUNDAY | Blueberry Muffins (page 114), Shake Template (page 107) | Rosemary Citrus Chicken (page 151), brown rice, Daily Salad (page 178) | Thai Basil Eggplant (page 195) |
| MONDAY | Shake Template (page 107) | Leftovers from Sunday | Avocado Spinach Pesto (page 218) served over pasta, Shredded Chicken (page 152) |
| TUESDAY | Blueberry Oatmeal Shake (page 110) | Leftovers from Monday | Rosemary Roasted Potatoes (page 166), Shredded Chicken (page 152), Steamed Broccoli (page 192) |
| WEDNESDAY | Basic Oatmeal (page 111) | Leftovers from Tuesday | Baked Trout with Fennel (page 144), brown rice |
| THURSDAY | Shake Template (page 107) | Leftovers from Wednesday | Shrimp and Spicy Rice Noodles (page 213) |
| FRIDAY | Beet Green Smoothie (page 109) | Leftovers from Thursday | Basil, Watermelon, Tomato Skewers (page 174), Baked Tofu (page 137), Artisan Bread (page 170) |
| SATURDAY | Cherry Chia Jam (page 128) on Artisan Bread (page 170) | Leftovers from Friday | Miso-Glazed Whitefish (page 149), Daily Salad (page 178), Black Rice Pilaf (page 171) |

## WEEK 2

| | BREAKFAST | LUNCH | DINNER |
|---|---|---|---|
| SUNDAY | Two-Ingredient Granola (page 118), Shake Template (page 107) | Gingered Collards (page 182), Baked Chicken (page 139), Black Rice Pilaf (page 171) | Rosemary Citrus Chicken (page 151), Gingered Collards (page 182), Black Rice Pilaf (page 171) |
| MONDAY | Shake Template (page 107) | Leftovers from Sunday | Seared Baby Bok Choy (page 183), Baked Tofu (page 137), brown rice |
| TUESDAY | Basic Oatmeal (page 111) | Leftovers from Monday | Creamy Broccoli Pistachio Soup (page 181), Artisan Bread (page 170), Baked Tofu (page 137) |
| WEDNESDAY | Shake Template (page 107) | Leftovers from Tuesday | Trout en Papillote (page 153), Daily Salad (page 178), brown rice |
| THURSDAY | Basic Oatmeal (page 111) | Leftovers from Wednesday | Rosemary Cauliflower Creamed Soup (page 191), Baked Chicken (page 139), brown rice |
| FRIDAY | Shake Template (page 107) | Leftovers from Thursday | Caramelized Onion Pudding (page 159), Baked Chicken (page 139) |
| SATURDAY | Blueberry Muffins (page 114), Shake Template (page 107) | Minestrone Meatloaf (page 211) | Lentil Veggie Soup (page 210) |

# Week 1 Shopping List (4 Adults)

## PANTRY STAPLES

### Spices

Black pepper

Cayenne pepper

Kosher salt

White pepper

### Condiments

Apple cider vinegar

Balsamic vinegar

Dijon mustard

Honey

Neutral cooking oil
(avocado, canola,
grapeseed)

Olive oil

Rice vinegar

Tamari soy sauce

Toasted sesame seed oil

### Others

All-purpose flour
(unbleached, unenriched)

Arrowroot/cornstarch

Baking powder
(aluminum free)

Basmati rice

Brown rice

Flax milk, unsweetened

Nutritional yeast
(folic acid free)

Rolled oats

Stevia

Sucanat

White cooking wine

Whole wheat flour

## NONPERISHABLES

1 pound whole almonds

1 (8-ounce) jar
unsweetened applesauce

1 (32-ounce) carton
chicken broth

1 (8-ounce) jar maple syrup

1 (14.5-ounce) can
navy beans

1 (12-ounce) package
rice noodles

Peanut butter, crunchy

Protein powder:
Top picks include pea or
soy protein with at least
22 grams of protein per
serving.

## PERISHABLES

### Produce

2 medium avocados

2 bunches fresh basil

1 bunch beets

1 pound frozen blueberries

1 (10- to 16-ounce) package
frozen mango

2 pounds carrots

1 pint cherry tomatoes

2 cucumbers

1 package frozen edamame
(without pods)

2 Japanese eggplants

4 servings fresh or frozen
fruit for shakes (bananas,
berries, or others)

1 bulb garlic

2 fresh jalapeño peppers

2 jicamas

3 lemons

1 (8-ounce) container
white button mushrooms

3 medium onions

1 bunch fresh oregano

3 pounds peaches

1 red bell pepper

1 bunch radishes

1 bunch fresh rosemary

1 bunch fresh scallions

10 ounces spinach leaves

1 small seedless watermelon

5 pounds chicken breast

1 dozen eggs

1 pound shrimp, frozen,
peeled, and deveined,
large (21 to 29 per pound)

1 (15-ounce) block
extra-firm tofu

3 pounds trout fillets

# Week 2 Shopping List (4 Adults)

## PANTRY STAPLES

### Spices

Black pepper

Cayenne pepper

Kosher salt

White pepper

### Condiments

Balsamic vinegar

Dijon mustard

Honey

Neutral cooking oil
(avocado, canola,
grapeseed)

Olive oil

Rice vinegar

Tamari soy sauce

Toasted sesame seed oil

### Others

All-purpose flour
(unbleached, unenriched)

Arrowroot/cornstarch

Baking powder
(aluminum-free)

Black rice

Bread flour

Brown rice

Flax milk, unsweetened

Nutritional yeast
(folic-acid free)

Rolled oats

Sesame seeds

Stevia

Sucanat

White cooking wine

Whole wheat flour

## NONPERISHABLES

1 pound whole almonds

1 (8-ounce) jar unsweetened applesauce

1 (3.5-ounce) jar capers

1 (32-ounce) carton chicken broth

1 (10-ounce) jar kalamata olives

1 (8-ounce) jar maple syrup

1 (8-ounce) package shelled pistachios

Protein powder: Top picks include pea or soy protein with at least 22 grams of protein per serving.

2 (32-ounce) cartons vegetable broth

## PERISHABLES

### Produce

2 pounds baby bok choy

1 green bell pepper

1 pound frozen blueberries

4 heads broccoli

1 pound carrots

1 pint cherry tomatoes

2 cucumbers

2 bunches collard greens

2 servings fresh or frozen fruit for shakes (bananas, berries, or others)

1 bulb garlic

¼ pound gingerroot

2 jicamas

2 lemons

6 medium onions

2 medium sweet onions,

1 bunch fresh oregano

1 bunch fresh parsley

1 bunch radishes

1 bunch fresh rosemary

10 ounces spinach leaves

### Protein and Dairy

8 pounds chicken breast

1 dozen eggs

6 ounces white miso paste

4 (15-ounce) blocks extra-firm tofu

2 pounds trout fillets

# Daily Notes for Week 2

### SUNDAY

Be sure to make a double batch of Black Rice Pilaf today. You can also make a larger batch and use it for Monday's dinner in place of brown rice.

### THURSDAY

Baked Chicken for tonight and tomorrow—be sure to do a double batch.

### SATURDAY

You're finished! Time to make your next plans. Another 14-Day Menu Plan? Repeat some favorites? Try recipes outside of a plan?

# 14-Day Menu Plan to Cool Down

*Featured Foods: Cabbage, Citrus, Figs, Soy, Turmeric*

## WEEK 1

| | BREAKFAST | LUNCH | DINNER |
|---|---|---|---|
| **SUNDAY** | Carob Fig Balls (page 124), Shake Template (page 107) | Seared Baby Bok Choy (page 183), Baked Chicken (page 139), millet | Creamy Shrimp and Tofu Soup (page 142) |
| **MONDAY** | Shake Template (page 107) | Leftovers from Sunday | Lemon Baked Chicken (page 143), Daily Salad (page 178), brown rice |
| **TUESDAY** | Basic Oatmeal (page 111) | Leftovers from Monday | Sesame Orange Chicken (page 134) |
| **WEDNESDAY** | Basic Oatmeal (page 111) | Leftovers from Tuesday | Lemony Cabbage Soup (page 187), Shredded Chicken (page 152), Artisan Bread (page 170) |
| **THURSDAY** | Shake Template (page 107) | Leftovers from Wednesday | Tofu Veggie Laksa (page 214), Steamed Broccoli (page 192), Kamut |
| **FRIDAY** | Turmeric Banana Shake (page 106) | Leftovers from Thursday | Curried Almond Squash Soup (page 179), Baked Chicken (page 139), Kamut |
| **SATURDAY** | Shake Template (page 107) | Leftovers from Friday | Lime-Sautéed Scallops (page 150), Steamed Broccoli (page 192), quinoa |

## WEEK 2

| | BREAKFAST | LUNCH | DINNER |
|---|---|---|---|
| SUNDAY | Oatmeal Fig Bars (page 116), Shake Template (page 107) | Minestrone Meatloaf (page 211) | Poached Trout (page 147), Seared Baby Bok Choy (page 183), quinoa |
| MONDAY | Shake Template (page 107) | Leftovers from Sunday | Fig Arugula Salad (page 176) topped with Shredded Chicken (page 152), Artisan Bread (page 170) |
| TUESDAY | Turmeric Banana Shake (page 106) | Leftovers from Monday | Sesame Coleslaw (page 194), Baked Chicken (page 139), Artisan Bread (page 170) |
| WEDNESDAY | Basic Oatmeal (page 111) | Leftovers from Tuesday | Foil-Baked Chicken and Radishes (page 206) |
| THURSDAY | Two-Ingredient Granola (page 118), Shake Template (page 107) | Leftovers from Wednesday | Sesame Orange Chicken (page 134) |
| FRIDAY | Shake Template (page 107) | Leftovers from Thursday | Lemon Baked Chicken (page 143), Roasted Root Veggies (page 190), Artisan Bread (page 170) |
| SATURDAY | Carob Fig Balls (page 124), Shake Template (page 107) | Artisan Bread (page 170), Fig Arugula Salad (page 176), leftover chicken | Curried Eggplant, Chickpeas, and Tomatoes (page 201) |

# Week 1 Shopping List (4 Adults)

## PANTRY STAPLES

### Spices

Black pepper

Cinnamon

Carob powder

Curry powder

Kosher salt

Red pepper flakes

Thai red chilis, dried

Vanilla extract

White pepper

### Condiments

Apple cider vinegar

Balsamic vinegar

Chili sauce

Honey

Maple syrup

Neutral cooking oil
(avocado, canola,
grapeseed)

Olive oil

Rice vinegar

Tamari soy sauce

Toasted sesame seed oil

### Others

All-purpose flour
(unbleached, unenriched)

Arrowroot/cornstarch

Baking powder
(aluminum-free)

Bread flour

Brown rice

Flax milk, unsweetened

Nutritional yeast
(folic acid free)

Rolled oats

Sesame seeds

Stevia

Sucanat

Whole wheat flour

## NONPERISHABLES

1 pound whole almonds

1 (32-ounce) carton chicken
broth

1 (8.5-ounce) can light
coconut milk

1 (10-ounce) jar kalamata
olives

8 ounces dried figs

1 pound whole grain Kamut

1 (8-ounce) jar maple syrup

1 pound whole grain millet

8 ounces shelled pistachios

Protein powder:
Top picks include pea or
soy protein with at least
22 grams of protein per
serving.

1 pound quinoa

1 (8-ounce) pack rice noodles

1 (4-ounce) can Thai red
curry paste

1 (15.5-ounce) can diced
tomatoes

1 (8-ounce) can tomato sauce

## PERISHABLES

### Produce

5 bunches baby bok choy

1 banana

1 bunch beets

1 pound frozen blueberries

3 heads broccoli

2 small heads cauliflower

1 pound carrots

1 pound baby carrots

1 head cauliflower

1 bunch celery stalks

1 pint cherry tomatoes

1 bunch cilantro

1 cucumber

4 servings fresh or frozen fruit for shakes (bananas, berries, or others)

3 bulbs garlic

¼ pound gingerroot

1 jicama

2 lemons

1 package fresh lemongrass

2 limes

1 (16-ounce) bag mung bean sprouts

16 ounces white button mushrooms

3 medium onions

1 bunch fresh oregano

1 bunch fresh parsley

1 bunch radishes

1 red bell pepper

1 bunch scallions

1 (8-ounce) bag snow peas

10 ounces spinach leaves

2 medium kabocha squash

1 pound zucchini

### Protein and Dairy

11 pounds chicken breast

1 dozen eggs

6 ounces white miso paste

1 pound frozen sea scallops

1 pound frozen shrimp

1 (15-ounce) block extra-firm tofu

1 (15-ounce) block soft tofu

# Daily Notes for Week 1

### SUNDAY

The Carob Fig Balls are great to have on hand. Feel free to make a larger batch to snack on for the future.

### THURSDAY

Make quadruple of the Kamut—we'll need some tomorrow and Saturday. Any other whole grain can work in its place as well.

### SATURDAY

Make a double batch of quinoa. Shopping day! Check your shopping list.

# Week 2 Shopping List (4 Adults)

## PANTRY STAPLES

### Spices

Bay leaves

Black pepper

Cayenne pepper

Cinnamon

Carob powder

Curry powder

Kosher salt

Oregano, dried

Red pepper flakes

Thyme, dried

Turmeric powder

### Condiments

Apple cider vinegar

Balsamic vinegar

Dijon mustard

Honey

Maple syrup

Neutral cooking oil
   (avocado, canola,
   grapeseed)

Olive oil

Rice vinegar

Tamari soy sauce

Toasted sesame oil

### Others

All-purpose flour
   (unbleached, unenriched)

Arrowroot/cornstarch

Baking soda

Bread flour

Flax milk, unsweetened

Nutritional yeast
   (folic-acid free)

Rolled oats

Sesame seeds

Stevia

Sucanat

Whole wheat flour

## NONPERISHABLES

1 pound whole almonds

1 (8-ounce) jar
   unsweetened applesauce

1 (14.5-ounce) can
   cannellini beans

1 (32-ounce) carton
   chicken broth

1 (14.5-ounce) can
   chickpeas

1 (8.5-ounce) can
   coconut milk

8 ounces dried figs

Protein powder:
   Top picks include pea
   or soy protein with at
   least 22 grams of protein
   per serving.

1 (15.5-ounce) can diced
   tomatoes

1 (4-ounce) can tomato paste

## PERISHABLES

### Produce

2 bunches arugula

2 pounds baby bok choy

1 banana

1 bunch beets

1 pound frozen blueberries

2 bunches broccoli

1 medium head cabbage

1 pound carrots

1 pint cherry tomatoes

1 bunch cilantro

1 cucumber

1 medium eggplant

4 servings fresh or frozen fruit for shakes (bananas, berries, or others)

3 bulbs garlic

¼ pound gingerroot

1 jicama

4 lemons

2 limes

2 medium onions

1 medium sweet onion

1 red onion

1 bunch fresh oregano

1 bunch fresh parsley

2 bunches radishes

2 pounds root veggies of choice (sweet potatoes, potatoes, turnips, parsnips, etc.)

1 bunch scallions

10 ounces spinach leaves

1 pound sweet potatoes

1 pound zucchini

### Protein and Dairy

9 pounds chicken breast

1 dozen eggs

6 ounces white miso paste

2 pounds trout fillets

2 pounds lean (90–97%) ground turkey

# Daily Notes for Week 2

## SUNDAY

Tomorrow's dinner will call for some bread. You can make it tomorrow or start it today if you'd like it to have an extra day to ferment.

## SATURDAY

You're finished! Time to make your next plans. Another 14-Day Menu Plan? Repeat some favorites? Try recipes outside of a plan?

# 14-Day Menu Plan for Better Sleep
*Featured Foods: Black Rice, Cherries, Kiwi, Pistachios, Poultry*

## WEEK 1

| | BREAKFAST | LUNCH | DINNER |
|---|---|---|---|
| SUNDAY | Easy Cherry Crumble (page 120), Shake Template (page 107) | Artisan Bread (page 170), Roasted Beet and Pistachio Salad (page 188), Shredded Chicken (page 152) | Rosemary Cherry Compote (page 129) over Shredded Chicken (page 152), Artisan Bread (page 170), Daily Salad (page 178) |
| MONDAY | Shake Template (page 107) | Leftovers from Sunday | Forbidden Tempeh Rice (page 198) |
| TUESDAY | Shake Template (page 107) | Leftovers from Monday | Baked Paprika Chicken with Brussels Sprouts (page 140) |
| WEDNESDAY | Basic Oatmeal (page 111) | Leftovers from Tuesday | Black Rice Pilaf (page 171), Poached Ginger Chicken (page 146), Steamed Broccoli (page 192) |
| THURSDAY | Shake Template (page 107) | Leftovers from Wednesday | Baked Tofu (page 137), Black Rice Pilaf (page 171), Daily Salad (page 178) |
| FRIDAY | Basic Oatmeal (page 111) | Leftovers from Thursday | Roasted Root Veggies (page 190), Baked Tofu (page 137), Steamed Broccoli (page 192) |
| SATURDAY | Shake Template (page 107) | Leftovers with Kiwi Cucumber Salad (page 186) | Baked Chicken (page 139), Kiwi Bread (page 115), Daily Salad (page 178) |

## WEEK 2

| | BREAKFAST | LUNCH | DINNER |
|---|---|---|---|
| SUNDAY | Kiwi Bread (page 115), Shake Template (page 107) | Ginger Garlic Stir-Fry (page 204) | Baked Chicken (page 139), Artisan Bread (page 170), Daily Salad (page 178) topped with Toasted Pistachios with Chili (page 228) |
| MONDAY | Shake Template (page 107) | Leftovers from Sunday | Creamy Broccoli Pistachio Soup (page 181), Baked Chicken (page 139), brown rice |
| TUESDAY | Shake Template (page 107) | Leftovers from Monday | Sesame Orange Chicken (page 134) |
| WEDNESDAY | Basic Oatmeal (page 111) | Leftovers from Tuesday | Baked Paprika Chicken with Brussels Sprouts (page 140) |
| THURSDAY | Kiwi Chia Pudding (page 131), Shake Template (page 107) | Leftovers from Wednesday | Roasted Beet and Pistachio Salad (page 188), Baked Tofu (page 137) |
| FRIDAY | Basic Oatmeal (page 111) | Leftovers from Thursday | Forbidden Tempeh Rice (page 198) |
| SATURDAY | Cherry Chia Jam (page 128), Artisan Bread (page 170) | Leftovers plus Kiwi Cucumber Salad (page 186) | Poached Ginger Chicken (page 146), Daily Salad (page 178) with Sesame Soy Dressing (page 223), brown rice |

# Week 1 Shopping List (4 Adults)

## PANTRY STAPLES

### Spices

Black pepper

Cumin, ground

Garlic salt

Italian seasoning

Kosher salt

Onion powder

Paprika

Red pepper flakes

### Condiments

Apple cider vinegar

Balsamic vinegar

Dijon mustard

Honey

Maple syrup

Neutral cooking oil
(avocado, canola,
grapeseed)

Olive oil

Rice vinegar

Tamari soy sauce

Toasted sesame oil

### Others

All-purpose flour
(unbleached, unenriched)

Arrowroot/cornstarch

Baking powder
(aluminum-free)

Baking soda

Bread flour

Black rice

Brown rice

Flax milk, unsweetened

Nutritional yeast
(folic acid free)

Rolled oats

Sesame seeds

Stevia

Sucanat

Walnuts

Whole wheat flour

## NONPERISHABLES

1 pound whole almonds

1 (8-ounce) jar
unsweetened applesauce

3 (14.5-ounce) can
cannellini beans

1 (32-ounce) carton
chicken broth

1 (14.5-ounce) can
chickpeas

1 (8.5-ounce) can
coconut milk

8 ounces dried figs

8 ounces shelled unsalted
pistachios

Protein powder:
Top picks include pea
or soy protein with at
least 22 grams of protein
per serving.

1 (8-ounce or larger)
container green chili salsa
(salsa verde)

1 (15.5-ounce) can diced
tomatoes

1 (4-ounce) can tomato paste

## PERISHABLES

### Produce

2 bunches arugula

1 pound baby bok choy

1 banana

2 bunches beets

1 head broccoli

1 pound Brussels sprouts

1 pound carrots

1 pint cherry tomatoes

1 bunch cilantro

3 cucumbers

1 English cucumber

1 medium eggplant

4 servings fresh or frozen fruit for shakes (bananas, berries, or others)

3 bulbs garlic

¼ pound gingerroot

1 pound green beans

2 jalapeño peppers

2 pounds kiwifruit

1 package lemongrass

1 bunch mint

2 (8-ounce) containers white button mushrooms

4 medium onions

1 bunch radishes

1 red bell pepper

1 bunch romaine lettuce

2 pounds root veggies of choice (sweet potatoes, potatoes, turnips, parsnips, etc.)

2 bunches scallions

1 medium shallot

10 ounces spinach leaves

### Protein and Dairy

9 pounds chicken breast

1 dozen eggs

1 (15-ounce) block extra-firm tofu

# Daily Notes for Week 1

### SUNDAY

Lots of cherry dishes today! Make a double batch of Shredded Chicken at lunch.

### WEDNESDAY

Be sure to do a double batch of Black Rice Pilaf.

### THURSDAY

Baked Tofu alert! Do a double batch so you have some ready for tomorrow.

### SATURDAY

When you peel and slice kiwi for today's salad, prep enough for tonight's bread as well. Shopping day! Check your shopping list.

# Week 2 Shopping List (4 Adults)

## PANTRY STAPLES

### Spices

Black pepper

Cumin, ground

Garlic salt

Italian seasoning

Kosher salt

Onion powder

Oregano, dried

Paprika

Red pepper flakes

### Condiments

Apple cider vinegar

Balsamic vinegar

Dijon mustard

Honey

Maple syrup

Neutral cooking oil
(avocado, canola,
grapeseed)

Olive oil

Rice vinegar

Tamari soy sauce

Toasted sesame oil

### Others

All-purpose flour
(unbleached, unenriched)

Arrowroot/cornstarch

Baking powder
(aluminum-free)

Baking soda

Bread flour

Black rice

Brown rice

Flax milk, unsweetened

Nutritional yeast
(folic-acid free)

Rolled oats

Sesame seeds

Stevia

Sucanat

Walnuts

Whole wheat flour

## NONPERISHABLES

1 pound whole almonds

1 (8-ounce) jar
unsweetened applesauce

1 pound chia seeds

1 (32-ounce) carton
chicken broth

1 (15.5-ounce) can cubed,
unsweetened pineapple

16 ounces unsalted,
shelled pistachios

Protein powder:
Top picks include pea
or soy protein with at
least 22 grams of protein
per serving.

1 (32-ounce) carton
vegetable broth

## PERISHABLES

### Produce

2 bunches beets

5 heads broccoli

1 pound Brussels sprouts

1 pound carrots

1 pound fresh or frozen cherries

1 bunch cilantro

1 cucumber

4 servings fresh or frozen fruit for shakes (bananas, berries, or others)

3 bulbs garlic

¼ pound gingerroot

1 pound green beans

3 jicamas

3 pounds kiwifruit

1 pack fresh lemongrass

3 limes

1 bunch mint

8 ounces white button mushrooms

3 medium onions

1 bunch radishes

1 bunch romaine lettuce

2 pounds root veggies of choice (sweet potatoes, potatoes, turnip, parsnips, etc.)

3 bunches scallions

1 (8-ounce) bag snow peas

10 ounces spinach leaves

### Protein and Dairy

10 pounds chicken breast

1 dozen eggs

2 (15-ounce) blocks extra-firm tofu

# Daily Notes for Week 2

## MONDAY

Be sure to make a double batch of rice so that you're set for tomorrow.

## SATURDAY

You're finished! Time to make your next plans. Another 14-Day Menu Plan? Repeat some favorites? Try recipes outside of a plan?

# CHAPTER 9

# Recipes

Here is what we've all been waiting for—time for the food! Before we dive in, I've got a few notes on common ingredients and cooking suggestions.

You should think about meals as a combination of three elements—veggies, protein, and good carbs. Fats are a healthy part of the diet, but they end up in meals without less forethought. Most high-protein foods also have fat, and oil is used in cooking.

Breakfast items have their own section, as do a few sauces and snacks, but most dishes are categorized as Protein, Healthy Carbs, or Veggies. Some recipes have elements of all three, and these are called Complete Meals.

## Ingredients and Cooking Tips

### COOKING OILS

My favorite cooking oils are those with a neutral flavor, high heat resistance, and generous amounts of phytonutrients. Top picks include avocado, canola, and grapeseed. Extra-virgin olive oil is great as well but should be used more for salads or as a finishing ingredient.

With good technique, one can use oil sparingly without compromising flavor or heat transfer. The trick is to heat your cooking surface, add the oil, let it cure, then start cooking. I use an oil misting bottle and refill it with my own oil. After heating a pan on medium high for 30 seconds or so, I'll mist it evenly.

If needed, I'll use a silicone cooking brush to even it out. Then I'll heat the oil another 30 seconds or so until it starts to shimmer. At that point, I'll adjust to the desired cooking temperature and start cooking.

The same technique works for baking sheets and pans. Just put them in the hot oven briefly, remove, add the oil, put them back in the oven for another few seconds, remove, and add food.

### SALT

Top picks for salt include kosher salt such as Diamond Crystal and Morton brands and finishing salt such as Maldon Sea Salt. Kosher salt is fluffier than table salt. Most recipes list salt by units of volume—often teaspoons or fractions of a teaspoon. I wrote these recipes assuming the use of kosher salt. Most recipes you will find elsewhere are written assuming table salt. You'll need to double the volume of kosher salt for them.

## SWEETENERS

You have several options for sweeteners. There is no evidence that naturally occurring sweeteners are harmful when used in amounts that make sense in the context of your diet and your body's needs. There are also none that can't be used in amounts above what is healthy.

My default choice is Sucanat brand unrefined sweetener. It is rich in accessory vitamins and minerals and has been proven to be gentler on blood sugar levels than other sweeteners.[1] It is worth mentioning that Sucanat is not a noncaloric sweetener like stevia or monk fruit (lo han guo). Like sugar, it has roughly 15 calories per teaspoon. Sucanat has a good taste without overpowering recipes. If needed, you can substitute any other natural sweetener for it such as raw sugar, turbinado sugar, or unrefined cane sugar.

Other good options include stevia and monk fruit. These can be found in powdered forms—most products will say how sweet they

are in proportion to table sugar. They are also available in liquid forms. These are quite concentrated and will require adjustments to baking recipes. Check the manufacturer's website for suggestions.

## GARLIC AND GINGER

Nearly all the recipes use at least one of these ingredients. It does feel virtuous to properly peel and mince them by hand, but the process can take a fair amount of time. High-quality minced ginger is available in most grocery stores; look for it in jars in the spices or Asian food section. I also like to keep peeled garlic in stock—you can find it with refrigerated produce.

The taste compromise from using these pre-prepped forms is minimal, if any, but the time savings really add up. I find myself more likely to use them more often and in healthier quantities when they take less effort.

## ORGANIC OR COMMERCIAL PRODUCE?

Don't stress over this one—I don't. When you dig deep, you will find there are no compelling reasons to choose one over the other. Organic produce still has pesticides, commercial produce may be more environmentally friendly, and it is great to support local farmers. Choose the freshest, most cost-effective product you can find.

# Miscellaneous Tips

## OVEN TEMPERATURE

Please invest in an oven thermometer. The temperature inside the oven may not be the same as the temperature you set it to. If you have a thermometer in your oven, you can catch the difference and adjust as needed. I've used seven different ovens to test these recipes. One of them was almost always perfect, but all the others were off—in many cases by a lot!

## COOKING MATERIALS

Many ask about the safest materials for use in the kitchen. There are valid concerns about chemicals leaching into food, especially from plastics and some metals. The other consideration I consider is usability. Some "safer" materials just don't work well.

For cookware and bakeware, your best bets are stainless steel, cast iron, and anodized aluminum. For prep ware like cutting boards, containers, and utensils, choose stainless steel, silicone, glass, and wood.

## FOOD THERMOMETER

It is also good to have a food thermometer in your kitchen. Several meat recipes specify a particular temperature. Food thermometers have a narrow metal probe you insert into the dish. They display the temperature at the end of the probe, which allows you to determine the temperature on the inside. Better food thermometers read quickly and accurately.

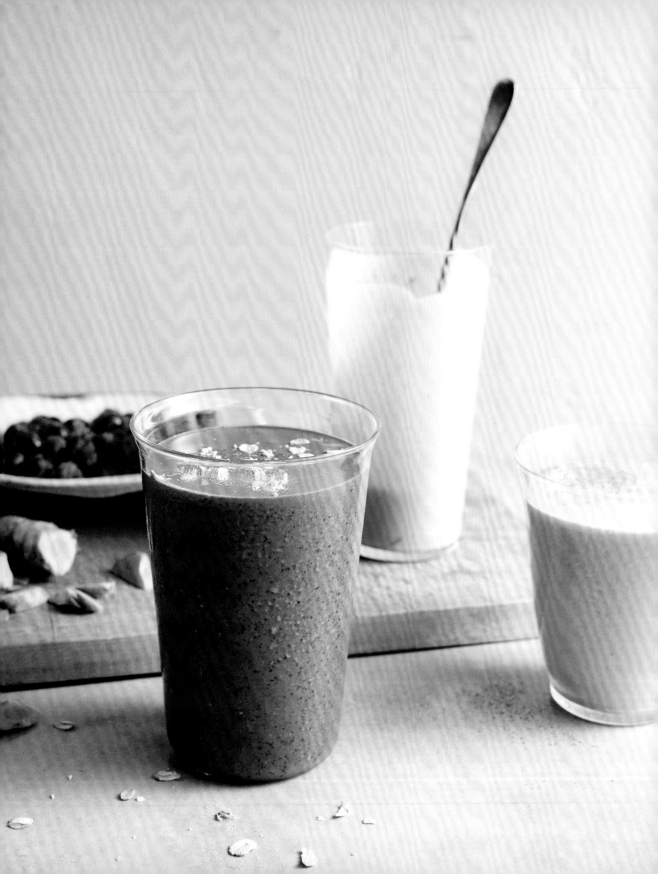

# Breakfast

The best place to start our recipes is with the first meal of the day. You have many types of options, including shakes, cereal dishes, and baked items (some of which can also be used for dessert). Many of these are easy to make the night before so that your morning is simple and stress-free.

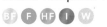
SYMPTOM KEY

- Brain fog
- Fatigue
- Hot flashes
- Insomnia
- Weight gain

# Turmeric Banana Shake

**SYMPTOMS IT CAN HELP**

**BF** Brain fog

**HF** Hot flashes

**I** Insomnia

**SERVES 1**
**Prep time:** 5 minutes
**Total time:** 5 minutes

**SERVING SUGGESTION**
Serve immediately for breakfast.

**RESET PHASE MODIFICATIONS**
**ADRENAL RESET**
**Meal:** Breakfast
**Modification:** None

**METABOLISM RESET**
**Meal:** Breakfast, lunch
**Modification:** None

**THYROID RESET**
**Meal:** Any
**Modification:** None

**GLUTEN-FREE OPTION**
No modification needed

**VEGAN OPTION**
No modification needed

Turmeric and banana combine to give this shake a beautiful color and rich flavor. The banana emulsifies the turmeric, hiding its bitter notes. Try to remember to use rubber gloves when handling fresh turmeric. Otherwise, if you're like me, you'll turn every fabric in sight yellow!

1 cup unsweetened flax milk

½ banana, peeled and frozen

½ teaspoon turmeric powder or 1 teaspoon fresh

1 serving protein powder, vanilla or unflavored

Optional: Stevia or another sweetener of choice to taste

- Add all the ingredients except protein powder to the bowl of a high-powered blender.

- Blend on high power for 2 minutes or until smooth.

- Add the protein powder and blend on low for just a few seconds until mixed.

# Shake Template

SYMPTOMS IT CAN HELP

BF Brain fog

F Fatigue

HF Hot flashes

I Insomnia

W Weight gain

SERVES 1
**Prep time:** 5 minutes
**Total time:** 5 minutes

SERVING SUGGESTION
Serve immediately for breakfast.

There are several specific shake recipes here and in my other books, but here is a guide you can use to make your own. Feel free to mix and match different ingredients based on what you have on hand.

1 cup liquid (top choices here include water, aquafaba, milk substitute, or milk—my favorite is unsweetened flax milk)

½ cup ice cubes

½ to 1 cup fresh or frozen fruit (best options include berries and bananas)

1 serving protein powder, vanilla or unflavored (I recommend pea or soy protein)

**OPTIONAL INCLUSIONS**

Use ¼ cup neutral thickener, like cooked navy beans or raw rolled oats. Omit if serving the shake with another dish containing carbs.

Greens like baby spinach leaves

Sweeteners like stevia, monk fruit, or xylitol

Flavor enhancers like carob powder, ground cinnamon, vanilla extract, or ginger

- Add all the ingredients except protein powder to the bowl of a high-powered blender. Blend on high power for 2 minutes or until smooth.

- Add the protein powder and blend on low for just a few seconds until mixed.

# Apple Almond Shake

F Fatigue

W Weight gain

SERVES 1
**Prep time:** 5 minutes
**Total time:** 5 minutes

SERVING SUGGESTION
Serve immediately for breakfast.

RESET PHASE
MODIFICATIONS
**ADRENAL RESET**
**Meal:** Breakfast, lunch
**Modification:** None

**METABOLISM RESET**
**Meal:** Breakfast, lunch
**Modification:** None

**THYROID RESET**
**Meal:** Any
**Modification:** None

GLUTEN-FREE OPTION
No modification needed

VEGAN OPTION
No modification needed

Here's one of our all-time favorite shake recipes. I like Granny Smith apples, but any kind of apple can work well.

¼ cup raw almonds

1 cup water

½ cup ice

1 Granny Smith apple, peeled and cored

½ teaspoon ground cinnamon

1 serving vegetable-based protein powder, vanilla or unflavored

Optional: Stevia, monk fruit, or other sweetener to taste

- Using a high-powered blender, blend the almonds into a fine flour. Add the water, ice, apple, and cinnamon and blend on high power for 1 minute until smooth.

- Add the protein powder and blend on low for just a few seconds until mixed. If the protein powder is unsweetened, add sweetener to taste.

# Beet Green Smoothie

**SYMPTOMS IT CAN HELP**

**BF** Brain fog

**F** Fatigue

**I** Insomnia

**SERVES 1**
**Prep time:** 5 minutes
**Total time:** 5 minutes

**SERVING SUGGESTION**
Serve immediately for breakfast.

**RESET PHASE MODIFICATIONS**
**ADRENAL RESET**
**Meal:** Breakfast, lunch
**Modification:** None

**METABOLISM RESET**
**Meal:** Breakfast, lunch
**Modification:** None

**THYROID RESET**
**Meal:** Any
**Modification:** None

**GLUTEN-FREE OPTION**
No modification needed

**VEGAN OPTION**
No modification needed

Beets usually come in a bunch, with the stems and greens attached. Beet greens are packed with vitamins and nutrients, so we're including them in this smoothie. I find it easiest to store fresh ginger in the freezer and grate as much as is needed with a Microplane. Once I finish, I put it back in the freezer.

1 cup water or unsweetened flax milk

1 cup loosely packed beet greens, stem included, washed and coarsely chopped

1 small to medium beet, washed and chopped into quarters

1 cup frozen mango

1 tablespoon lime juice

1 serving protein powder, vanilla or unflavored

Optional: Stevia, monk fruit, or other sweetener to taste

- Add all the ingredients except the protein powder to the bowl of a high-powered blender.

- Blend on high power for 2 minutes or until smooth.

- Add the protein powder and blend on low for just a few seconds until mixed.

# Blueberry Oatmeal Shake

**SERVES 1**
**Prep time:** 5 minutes
**Total time:** 5 minutes

**SERVING SUGGESTION**
Serve immediately for
breakfast.

**RESET PHASE
MODIFICATIONS**
**ADRENAL RESET**
**Meal:** Breakfast, lunch
**Modification:** None

**METABOLISM RESET**
**Meal:** Breakfast, lunch
**Modification:** None

**THYROID RESET**
**Meal:** Any
**Modification:** None

**GLUTEN-FREE OPTION**
No modification needed

**VEGAN OPTION**
No modification needed

Blueberries are a classic addition to oatmeal. Here is a way to have this same combo in a fast, high-protein breakfast. If you are using old-fashioned oats, blend them alone for 30 seconds first for more finely ground oats.

1 cup unsweetened
flax milk

1 cup fresh or frozen
blueberries

¼ cup rolled oats

1 serving protein
powder, vanilla or
unflavored

Optional: Stevia,
monk fruit, or other
sweetener to taste

- Add all the ingredients except the protein powder to the bowl of a high-powered blender.

- Blend on high power for 2 minutes or until smooth.

- Add the protein powder and blend on low for just a few seconds until mixed.

# Basic Oatmeal

SYMPTOMS IT CAN HELP

**BF** Brain fog

**F** Fatigue

**W** Weight gain

**SERVES 4**
**Prep time:** 3 minutes
**Total time:** 20 minutes

Oatmeal has been one of my breakfast staples for most of my life. Once you get the mixture boiling well, it takes very little heat to keep it cooking without boiling over. If your stove does not have a low enough setting, you can move the pan so only part of it is over the heat. Even if you are cooking for one, it is easy to make all 4 servings at once and refrigerate the rest for later.

2 cups old-fashioned rolled oats

4 cups water

**OPTIONAL TOPPINGS**

1 serving protein powder, vanilla or unflavored

½ cup blueberries

½ small apple, diced

1 tablespoon ground flaxseed

½ teaspoon ground cinnamon

Stevia, monk fruit, or other sweetener to taste

- Combine the rolled oats and water in a medium saucepan. Over medium heat, bring to a simmer while stirring. Turn the heat to its lowest setting, cover the pan, and let cook for 5 minutes.

- Remove from the heat and let sit an additional 5 minutes.

- Add a serving of protein powder either stirred into the oats or mixed in water as a drink.

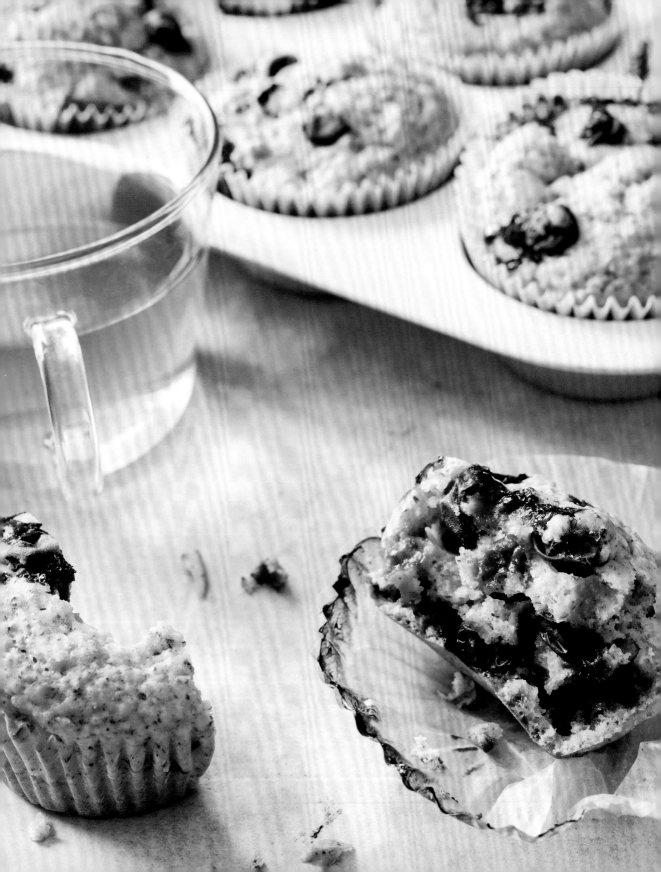

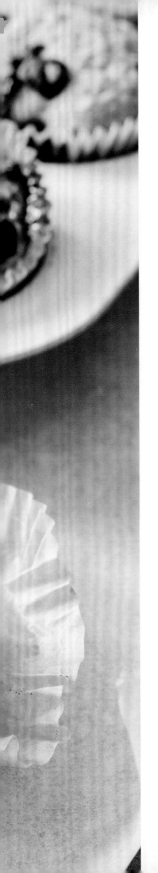

# BAKED BREAKFAST

On pages 114-123 and 126, you'll find some baked breakfast recipes that you can make in advance to save yourself some time on busy mornings. Bake them up the night before or during your food prep session. After cooling, they will keep for up to 5 days in a bread box or airtight container with some paper towels to absorb moisture.

# Blueberry Muffins

 Brain fog

 Insomnia

 Weight gain

**MAKES 12 MUFFINS**
**Prep time:** 15 minutes
**Total time:** 40 minutes

SERVING SUGGESTION
These can also be served as a snack or for the carbs at the main meal.

RESET PHASE MODIFICATIONS
**ADRENAL RESET**
**Meal:** Breakfast, lunch
**Modification:** Serve in place of other sources of carbs.

**METABOLISM RESET**
**Meal:** Dinner
**Modification:** Serve in place of other sources of carbs.

**THYROID RESET**
**Meal:** Any
**Modification:** None

GLUTEN-FREE OPTION
Use a gluten-free all-purpose flour like Bob's Red Mill.

VEGAN OPTION
Omit the egg whites and use an additional 1 tablespoon of ground flaxseed.

These are much lighter and less sweet than typical blueberry muffins. They can even work as a side dish for a meal. I like muffin cup liners made from parchment paper because they don't stick to the muffins. If you don't have oat flour on hand, you can blend rolled oats in a blender until they are broken down to a flour-like consistency. Don't stir much after adding blueberries, as it will turn the batter blue.

| | | |
|---|---|---|
| 1 cup all-purpose flour | 2 tablespoons ground flaxseed | ¼ cup liquid egg whites |
| ¾ cup oat flour | 2 tablespoons Sucanat or natural sweetener of choice | ½ cup unsweetened flax milk or milk of choice |
| 2 teaspoons aluminum-free baking powder | ½ cup unsweetened applesauce | 1 cup fresh or frozen blueberries |

- Preheat the oven to 350°F. Line 12 muffin cups with parchment muffin liners.

- Whisk together the flours, baking powder, flaxseed, and Sucanat in a medium bowl.

- In a separate bowl, stir together the applesauce, egg whites, and milk. Stir the flour mixture into the liquid ingredients, leaving a few streaks of flour. Carefully fold in the blueberries.

- Fill each cup in a muffin pan two-thirds full of the batter. Bake for 25 minutes, or until the muffins are a light tan on top. Let cool for 10 minutes before serving.

# Kiwi Bread

**SYMPTOMS IT CAN HELP**

BF Brain fog

F Fatigue

I Insomnia

**SERVES 12**
**Prep time:** 15 minutes
**Total time:** 55 minutes

**SERVING SUGGESTION**
Use this as a healthy carb
with any meal.

**RESET PHASE
MODIFICATIONS**
**ADRENAL RESET**
**Meal:** Any
**Modification:** None

**METABOLISM RESET**
**Meal:** Dinner
**Modification:** Serve with
veggies and protein.

**THYROID RESET**
**Meal:** Any
**Modification:** None

**GLUTEN-FREE OPTION**
Use a gluten-free
all-purpose flour like
Bob's Red Mill.

**VEGAN OPTION**
Omit the egg whites and
add ¼ cup of flaxseed
mixed into ¼ cup of
water; omit the milk and
use a plant-based milk.

You've heard about banana bread and zucchini bread. Here is a fresh new twist with a citrusy taste and vibrant color. Try it and you'll wonder why most recipes insist on using so much butter in fruit breads. White whole wheat flour is flour from a strain of wheat berry that is naturally lighter in color. You can use regular whole wheat flour instead, but it will be heavier.

Misting oil

1 cup all-purpose flour

½ cup white whole wheat flour

2 teaspoons baking powder

½ teaspoon kosher salt

½ cup Sucanat or natural sweetener of choice

¼ cup unsweetened applesauce

4 egg whites

½ cup skim milk or milk substitute

1 cup peeled and pureed kiwifruit (about 5)

- Preheat the oven to 350°F. Mist the oil into an 8×4-inch loaf pan.

- In a medium mixing bowl, combine the flours, baking powder, salt, and Sucanat.

- In another mixing bowl, combine the applesauce, egg whites, milk, and kiwifruit. Fold the dry mixture into the wet until just mixed.

- Spread the batter into the prepared pan. Bake for 40 minutes, until the top is lightly browned.

- Cool for 15 minutes and serve.

# Oatmeal Fig Bars

## SYMPTOMS IT CAN HELP

HF Hot flashes

I Insomnia

W Weight gain

## SERVES 12
**Prep time:** 30 minutes
**Total time:** 60 minutes

## RESET PHASE MODIFICATIONS

**ADRENAL RESET**
**Meal:** Lunch, dinner
**Modification:** Serve in place of other carbs.

**METABOLISM RESET**
**Meal:** Dinner
**Modification:** For occasional use, serve in place of other carbs.

**THYROID RESET**
**Meal:** Any
**Modification:** None

## GLUTEN-FREE OPTION
Use gluten-free oats.

## VEGAN OPTION
Omit the egg whites and add ¼ cup of flaxseed mixed into ¼ cup of water.

This is my favorite portable food to power long hikes. These bars are also great for an energy boost during the day. If you are lucky enough to have fresh figs, they can work as well; just reduce the water to ½ cup. This one is a little more work than many of the other recipes, but these bars will keep for up to 5 days if refrigerated.

Oat flour is available for purchase, but I don't use it often enough to keep it in stock. I use a food processor for this dish. First, I put in the 1½ cups of oats and process until it is almost as fine as flour. Then I add the rest of the dry ingredients, pulse a few more times, add the rest, and let it mix.

Misting oil

2 cups dried figs (about 12 ounces)

1 cup water

1 tablespoon lemon zest

¼ cup pure maple syrup

1½ cups oat flour

1 cup rolled oats

½ teaspoon baking soda

½ teaspoon kosher salt

1 teaspoon vanilla extract

2 egg whites

¼ cup unsweetened applesauce

- Preheat the oven to 350°F and mist the oil into an an 8-inch square baking dish.

- Cut off and discard the stems off the dried figs, cut them into quarters, and place in a small saucepan with the water and the lemon zest. Bring to a low boil over medium-high heat, then reduce to a simmer for 30 minutes. Remove from heat and cool for 10 minutes.

- Once cooled, transfer to the bowl of a blender or food processor. Add the maple syrup and blend until pureed into a paste.

- Combine the oat flour, rolled oats, baking soda, and salt in a bowl and mix thoroughly.

■ In a separate bowl, combine the vanilla, egg whites, and applesauce and stir. Add the dry ingredients to the wet and stir until lightly combined. Pour half of the batter into the baking dish. Use a spatula to smooth into an even bottom layer.

■ Scoop up the fig paste and spread it evenly over the bottom layer of batter. Spread the remaining batter evenly on top.

■ Bake for 25 to 30 minutes, until golden brown. Remove from the oven and let cool completely. Cut into 12 bars and store in an airtight container in the refrigerator.

# Two-Ingredient Granola

**F** Fatigue

**I** Insomnia

**W** Weight gain

**SERVES 6**
**Prep time:** 3 minutes
**Total time:** 15 minutes

**SERVING SUGGESTION**
Serve with protein for breakfast.

**RESET PHASE MODIFICATIONS**
**ADRENAL RESET**
**Meal:** Any
**Modification:** Serve in place of all other sources of carbs.

**METABOLISM RESET**
**Meal:** Dinner
**Modification:** Not a common dinner food, but it can be used. Include protein and serve in place of all other sources of carbs.

**THYROID RESET**
**Meal:** Any
**Modification:** None

**GLUTEN-FREE OPTION**
Use gluten-free rolled oats.

**VEGAN OPTION**
No modification needed

You're going to love this one! I love oats and I love crunch, so granola is a natural winner. Yet all the commercial ones are full of empty calories from oil and sugar. After countless unsatisfactory versions, here is the pinnacle of clean, healthy, tasty, and easy granola. It works best with maple syrup, but you can also use honey. If you like clusters in your granola, the trick is not to stir it at all. Spread it out on the baking sheet, bake, and let cool completely before putting it in a container.

3 cups rolled oats

½ cup maple syrup

Optional: ½ teaspoon kosher salt

- Preheat the oven to 375°F.

- In a medium bowl, mix all the ingredients well. Spread out on a baking sheet and bake for 10 minutes. Let cool and serve.

# Savory Spicy Granola

SYMPTOMS IT CAN HELP

Oats can also be used in savory dishes. This savory granola is versatile. It can be a travel snack or a breakfast when served with a protein shake, or it can be used like seasoned croutons on a salad!

**SYMPTOMS IT CAN HELP**

(BF) Brain fog

(F) Fatigue

(W) Weight gain

**SERVES 6**
**Prep time:** 3 minutes
**Total time:** 15 minutes

**SERVING SUGGESTION**
Serve with protein for breakfast.

**RESET PHASE MODIFICATIONS**
**ADRENAL RESET**
**Meal:** Breakfast
**Modification:** None

**METABOLISM RESET**
**Meal:** Dinner
**Modification:** Serve in place of all other sources of carbs and fat.

**THYROID RESET**
**Meal:** Any
**Modification:** None

**GLUTEN-FREE OPTION**
Use gluten-free rolled oats.

**VEGAN OPTION**
Omit the egg whites.

3 cups rolled oats

⅓ cup maple syrup

1 teaspoon garlic powder

1 teaspoon paprika

¼ teaspoon cayenne pepper

2 egg whites

¼ cup raw sunflower seeds

Kosher salt and freshly ground black pepper to taste

- Preheat the oven to 375°F.

- In a medium bowl, mix all the ingredients well. Spread out on a baking sheet and bake for 10 minutes. Let cool and serve.

# Easy Cherry Crumble

SYMPTOMS IT CAN HELP

BF Brain fog

F Fatigue

I Insomnia

**SERVES 4**
**Prep time:** 5 minutes
**Total time:** 45 minutes

SERVING SUGGESTION
Serve as dessert or in
place of carbs with a
meal.

RESET PHASE
MODIFICATIONS
**ADRENAL RESET**
**Meal:** Any
**Modification:** None

**METABOLISM RESET**
**Meal:** Dinner
**Modification:** Serve
with protein and veggies
without additional carbs
or fat.

**THYROID RESET**
**Meal:** Any
**Modification:** None

GLUTEN-FREE OPTION
Use gluten-free oats and
a gluten-free all-purpose
flour like Bob's Red Mill.

VEGAN OPTION
Use milk substitute.

Try to find frozen dark sweet cherries for this recipe, as they work great without any additional sweetener. Most other frozen cherries are tart. If these are what you have, you may want to use the optional honey. Fresh cherries work great when they are in season. You just have to pit them. If cherries are not available, this recipe can also be made with any kind of berry or cold-weather fruit. The ingredient list is short, and the process is easy!

Misting oil

⅓ cup all-purpose flour

¼ cup rolled oats

1 teaspoon baking powder

½ teaspoon kosher salt

½ cup skim milk or milk substitute

2 cups cherries

Optional:
¼ cup honey

- Preheat the oven to 400°F and lightly mist an 8-inch square baking pan with the oil.

- In a medium bowl, combine the flour, oats, baking powder, and salt and mix well. Stir the milk into the dry ingredients. Stop stirring before the flour mixture is completely combined.

- Pour the cherries into the baking pan and pour the batter on top of the cherries. Bake for 40 minutes or until lightly browned.

- Cool and serve.

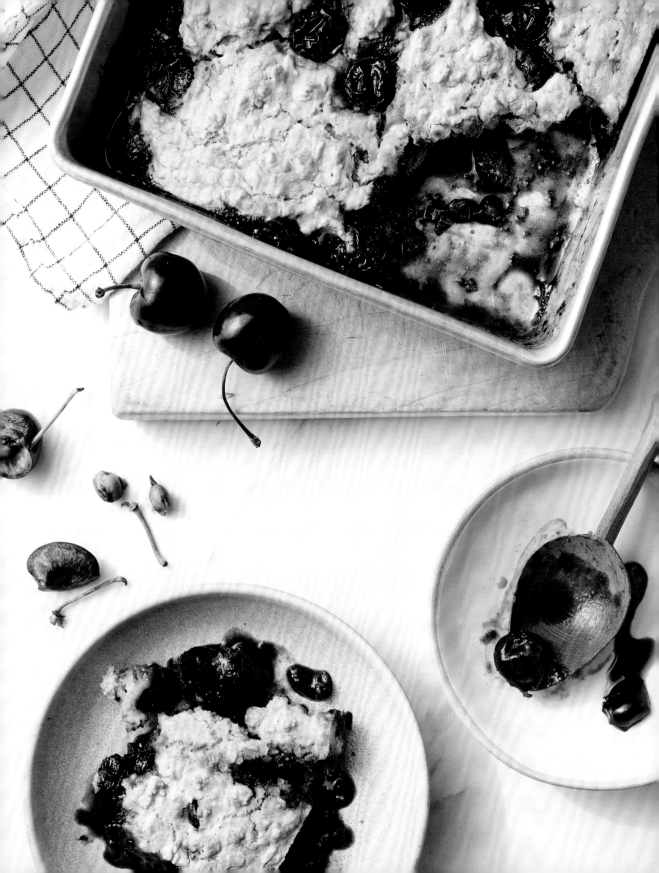

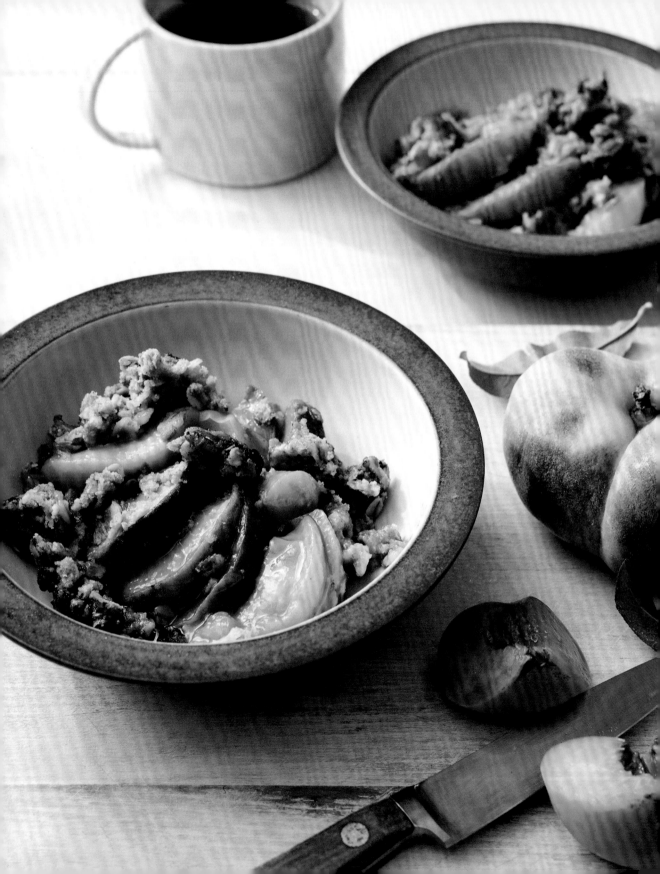

# Peach Walnut Cobbler

## SYMPTOMS IT CAN HELP

**BF** Brain fog

**F** Fatigue

**I** Insomnia

## SERVES 8
**Prep time:** 10 minutes
**Total time:** 1 hour and 20 minutes

## SERVING SUGGESTION
Use this as a good carb with any meal.

## RESET PHASE MODIFICATIONS
**ADRENAL RESET**
**Meal:** Any
**Modification:** Serve in place of all other sources of carbs and fat.

**METABOLISM RESET**
**Meal:** Dinner
**Modification:** Serve in place of all other sources of carbs and fat.

**THYROID RESET**
**Meal:** Any
**Modification:** None

## GLUTEN-FREE OPTION
Use gluten-free oats and a gluten-free all-purpose flour like Bob's Red Mill.

## VEGAN OPTION
No modification needed

Here is a good way to make use of fresh peaches when they all go ripe at once. Frozen peaches work fine as well. You don't need to adjust the cooking time.

Misting oil

¼ cup white whole wheat flour

2 tablespoons butter substitute spread (Smart Balance or Earth Balance brands)

½ cup rolled oats

½ cup chopped walnuts

⅓ cup Sucanat or natural sweetener of choice

1 teaspoon kosher salt

2½ pounds ripe peaches, pitted and thinly sliced

1 tablespoon lemon juice

■ Preheat the oven to 350°F and mist the oil into an 8×4-inch loaf pan.

■ In a medium bowl, mix the flour, spread, oats, walnuts, Sucanat, and salt. Combine the peaches and the lemon juice and distribute over the bottom of the prepared pan. Spread the cobbler mixture on top of the peaches.

■ Bake for 60 minutes, or until the fruit is tender and the top is lightly browned. Cool for 15 minutes and serve.

# Carob Fig Balls

SYMPTOMS IT CAN HELP

(F) Fatigue

(HF) Hot flashes

(I) Insomnia

**SERVES 12**
**Prep time:** 5 minutes
**Total time:** 5 minutes

**SERVING SUGGESTION**
Serve with a protein
shake for breakfast.

**RESET PHASE
MODIFICATIONS**
**ADRENAL RESET**
**Meal:** Lunch, dinner
**Modification:** Serve in
place of carbs and fat,
include protein.

**METABOLISM RESET**
**Meal:** Avoid
**Modification:** N/A

**THYROID RESET**
**Meal:** Any
**Modification:** None

**GLUTEN-FREE OPTION**
No modification needed

**VEGAN OPTION**
No modification needed

This recipe capitalizes on the phytonutrients found in figs. I prefer to use Calimyrna figs, as they have a more neutral flavor, but I have made it with Black Mission figs, and they still work. Use this dish as a breakfast for special occasions or as food to help fuel your next long hike. You can use any nuts or seeds in place of almonds without much change to the flavor.

1½ cups dried figs, stems removed (about 16 ounces)

½ cup whole almonds

⅓ cup carob powder

1 teaspoon vanilla extract

½ teaspoon ground cinnamon

½ teaspoon kosher salt

Optional: All-purpose flour for dusting

- Place the figs in a medium bowl, cover with hot water, and let them sit for 5 to 10 minutes.

- Pulse the almonds in the bowl of a food processor until they form a coarse meal. Add in the carob powder, vanilla, cinnamon, and salt.

- Drain the figs, then add to the food processor along with the almond mixture. Process all the ingredients until a dough forms.

- Roll out balls, each using 1 to 2 tablespoons of dough. Use a light dusting of flour if needed to keep them separated.

- Store in an airtight container in the fridge for up to 2 weeks, or in the freezer for up to 3 months.

# Cayenne Scrambled Eggs

BF Brain fog

F Fatigue

W Weight gain

**SERVES 4**
**Prep time:** 5 minutes
**Total time:** 12 minutes

**SERVING SUGGESTION**
Serve as part of one's
protein for breakfast.

**RESET PHASE
MODIFICATIONS**
**ADRENAL RESET**
**Meal:** Any
**Modification:** With
½ serving good carbs for
lunch, 1 serving for dinner

**METABOLISM RESET**
**Meal:** Dinner
**Modification:** With good
carbs, 1 serving

**THYROID RESET**
**Meal:** Any
**Modification:** For Reset
Phase, omit whole
eggs and use 12 egg
whites or 2 cups of Egg
Beaters egg substitute.
For maintenance phase,
whole eggs are fine.

**GLUTEN-FREE OPTION**
No modification needed

**VEGAN OPTION**
Use vegan egg replacer or
¾ cup chopped firm tofu.

This is a great quick breakfast when you're in the mood for eggs. They are good for the occasional option, but I don't make eggs a daily staple because they are too low in protein. Each egg contains only about 6 grams of protein, and each egg white has only 3 grams. If you are working hard to improve your protein status, have these as a side dish with a breakfast shake.

2 eggs

8 egg whites

4 tablespoons water

1 garlic clove,
minced

½ teaspoon
cayenne pepper

1 teaspoon
kosher salt

Misting oil

■ Combine all the ingredients except the oil in a medium bowl and whisk thoroughly.

■ Lightly mist a skillet with the oil and heat on high until the oil just starts to smoke. Reduce the heat to medium-high.

■ Pour the egg mixture into the pan and stir constantly for 2 to 3 minutes, or until the eggs are barely solid. Serve immediately.

# Spiced Banana Bread

## SYMPTOMS IT CAN HELP

**BF** Brain fog

**F** Fatigue

**W** Weight gain

## SERVES 12
**Prep time:** 15 minutes
**Total time:** 40 minutes

## SERVING SUGGESTION
Use this bread as a
dessert or a healthy carb.

## RESET PHASE
## MODIFICATIONS
**ADRENAL RESET**
**Meal:** Any
**Modification:** In place
of other carbs as an
occasional option—include
a source of protein.

**METABOLISM RESET**
**Meal:** Dinner
**Modification:** In place
of other carbs as an
occasional option—include
a source of protein.

**THYROID RESET**
**Meal:** Any
**Modification:** None

## GLUTEN-FREE OPTION
Use gluten-free oats and
a gluten-free all-purpose
flour like Bob's Red Mill.

## VEGAN OPTION
Omit the egg whites and
use 1 tablespoon
of ground flaxseed.

People are often surprised to find out how well cayenne pepper can work in desserts! Try it once as written below with ½ teaspoon of cayenne, and then feel free to adjust the amount of cayenne upward. I like to use a full teaspoon. Do stick with the same brand of cayenne. If you change brands, the heat level can change significantly.

Misting oil

2 egg whites

1 cup mashed banana (about 2 ripe bananas)

¼ cup unsweetened applesauce

1 cup all-purpose flour

½ cup rolled oats

½ cup Sucanat or natural sweetener of choice

1½ teaspoons aluminum-free baking powder

½ teaspoon baking soda

½ teaspoon cayenne pepper

- Preheat the oven to 350°F. Lightly mist the oil into a 8 × 4-inch loaf pan.

- In a medium bowl, mix the egg whites, mashed bananas, and applesauce.

- In a separate medium bowl, whisk together the flour, oats, Sucanat, baking powder, baking soda, and cayenne. Stir the flour mixture into the wet ingredients.

- Pour the batter into the loaf pan. Bake for 50 minutes, or until light tan on top and internal temperature is 200°F to 205°F.

- Let cool for 10 minutes before serving.

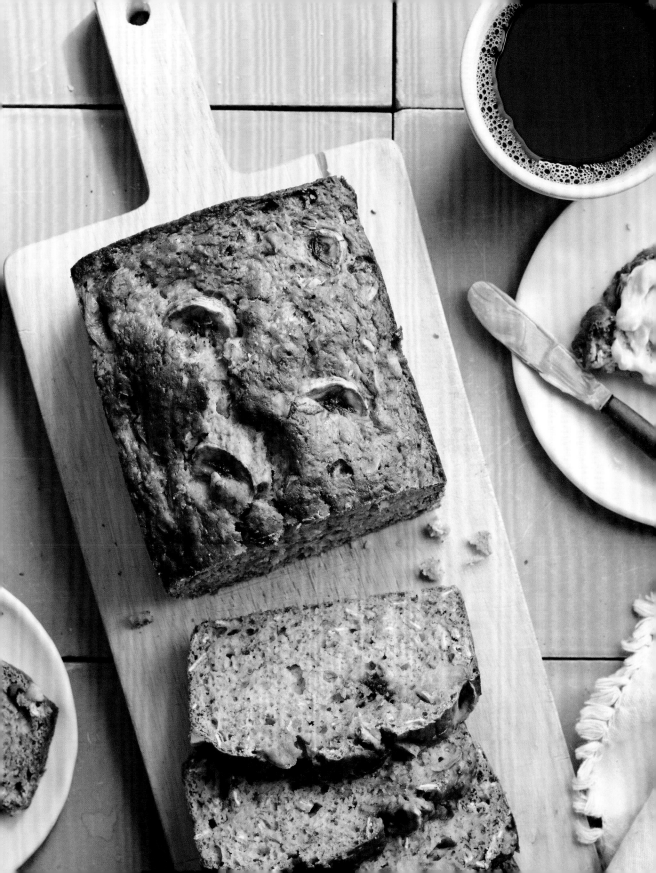

# Cherry Chia Jam

SERVES 16
**Prep time:** 5 minutes
**Total time:** 12 hours

SERVING SUGGESTION
Because this dish is high in healthy fats, if weight loss is an issue for you, leave out the fats from the meal you are pairing it with.

RESET PHASE
MODIFICATIONS
**ADRENAL RESET**
**Meal:** Any
**Modification:** Serve in place of all other sources of fat.

**METABOLISM RESET**
**Meal:** Dinner
**Modification:** Serve in place of all other sources of fat.

**THYROID RESET**
**Meal:** Any
**Modification:** None

GLUTEN-FREE OPTION
No modification needed

VEGAN OPTION
No modification needed

Here is an excellent topping for hot cereal or homemade bread. You might be amazed at how easy it is to make healthy jam! Either fresh or frozen can work for the cherries. For the pineapple you can use fresh, frozen, or canned—just be sure it is unsweetened.

| 2 cups pitted cherries | 1 cup pineapple cubes | 2 tablespoons chia seeds |
|---|---|---|

- Put the cherries and pineapple in a small saucepan. Cook over medium heat for 10 minutes, stirring constantly and mashing with a potato masher.

- Pour through a coarse colander to remove any large chunks of pineapple. Reserve the chunks for other uses, like adding to smoothies.

- Add in the chia seeds and mix well. Transfer the jam into a mason jar and refrigerate overnight.

# Rosemary Cherry Compote

## SYMPTOMS IT CAN HELP

**BF** Brain fog

**F** Fatigue

**I** Insomnia

**SERVES 8**
**Prep time:** 5 minutes
**Total time:** 45 minutes

**SERVING SUGGESTION**
Add to chicken or
seafood as a sauce.

**RESET PHASE
MODIFICATIONS**
**ADRENAL RESET**
**Meal:** Any
**Modification:** None

**METABOLISM RESET**
**Meal:** Dinner
**Modification:** Serve with
protein and veggies and
without additional fat.

**THYROID RESET**
**Meal:** Any
**Modification:** None

**GLUTEN-FREE OPTION**
No modification needed

**VEGAN OPTION**
No modification needed

When you find a nice crop of cherries, pit them all, use a batch or two for this recipe, and freeze the rest for shakes. This compote will keep in the refrigerator for several weeks and can be used to make a basic poultry or tofu dish exceptional! If needed, you can use onion in place of the shallots and water in place of the cherry juice.

Misting oil

2 tablespoons minced shallots (1 medium shallot)

2½ cups pitted sweet cherries, quartered (roughly 1 pound unpitted cherries)

¼ cup chopped walnuts

¼ cup cherry juice

1 tablespoon honey

½ teaspoon dried rosemary

Kosher salt and freshly ground black pepper to taste

- Mist a frying pan with the oil and heat on medium-high until the oil shimmers.

- Sauté the shallots, stirring frequently, for 2 to 3 minutes, or until softened. Stir in the cherries and the walnuts. Lower the heat to medium and stir for 4 to 5 minutes, until the cherries are soft.

- Add the cherry juice, honey, rosemary, salt, and pepper, mix thoroughly, and reduce the heat to low. Let cook for 30 minutes uncovered, stirring occasionally.

- Taste and add salt if needed. Let sit for at least 15 minutes so the flavors can meld.

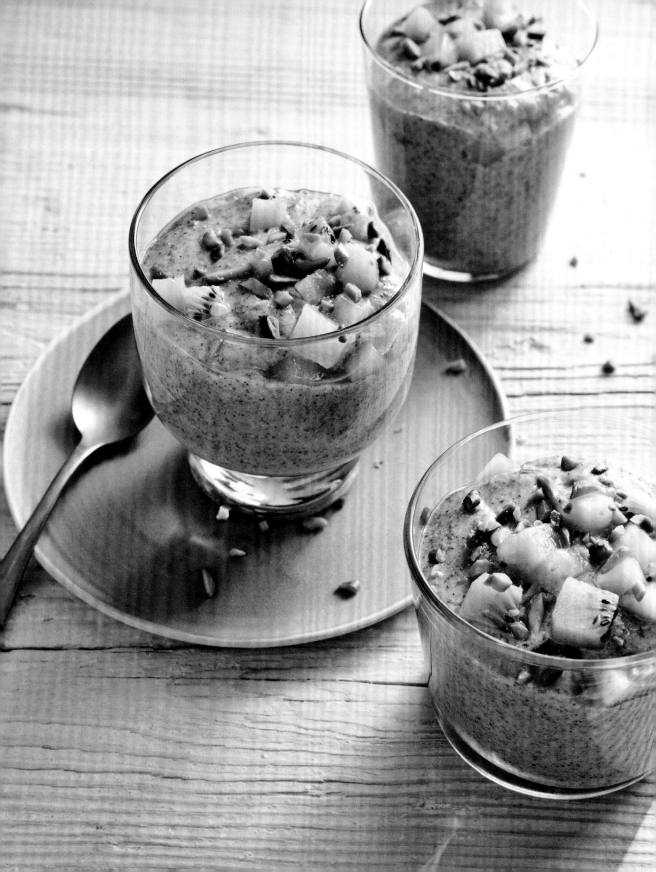

# Kiwi Chia Pudding

**SYMPTOMS IT CAN HELP**

F  Fatigue

HF  Hot flashes

I  Insomnia

**SERVES 4**
**Prep time:** 3 minutes
**Total time:** 5 minutes

**SERVING SUGGESTION**
Because this dish is high in healthy fats, if weight loss is an issue for you, leave out the fats from the meal you are pairing this with.

**RESET PHASE MODIFICATIONS**
**ADRENAL RESET**
**Meal:** Any
**Modification:** None

**METABOLISM RESET**
**Meal:** Dinner
**Modification:** Serve with carbs, veggies, and protein and without additional fat.

**THYROID RESET**
**Meal:** Any
**Modification:** None

**GLUTEN-FREE OPTION**
No modification needed

**VEGAN OPTION**
No modification needed

Chia pudding is better than Jell-O because it can work with acidic fruit. I especially like to use golden kiwi for this dish. They have the same nutritional benefits as green kiwi but a more subtle flavor.

3 tablespoons chia seeds

1 cup unsweetened flax milk

1 tablespoon maple syrup

1 teaspoon vanilla extract

1 cup kiwi, peeled and diced (about 3 fruits)

2 tablespoons chopped pistachios

- Add all the ingredients except the pistachios to the bowl of a blender and blend for 1 to 2 minutes, until smooth.

- Pour into a bowl, cover, and refrigerate at least 1 hour. Garnish with chopped pistachios and enjoy!

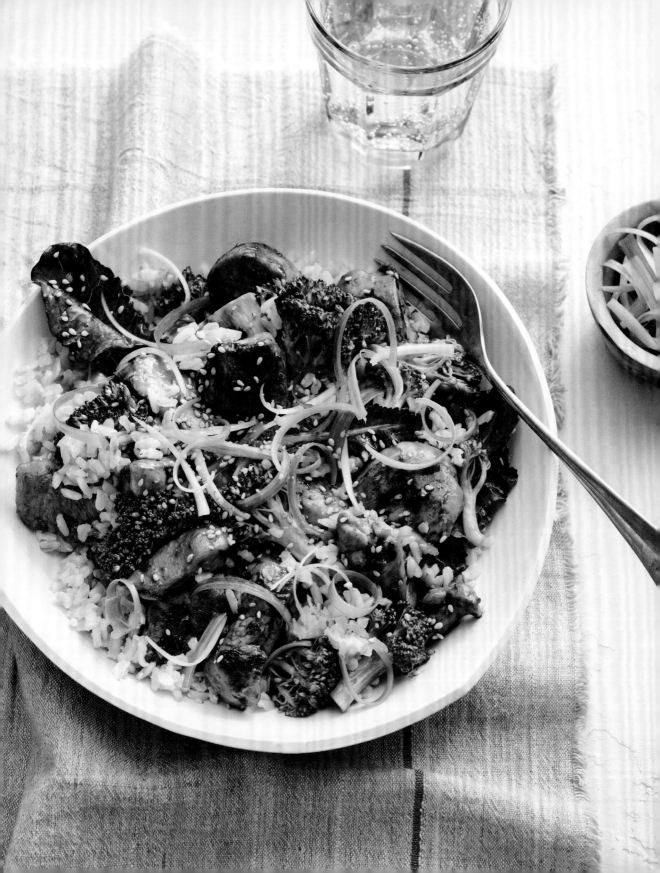

# Protein

When building a meal, think about protein, carbs, and veggies as the main building blocks. The best visual proportions for the plate are roughly ¼ carbs, ¼ protein, and ½ veggies.

Protein is worth special consideration because many find it can be the solution to troublesome symptoms. The truth is, people do not get protein deficient, but that fact shouldn't lead us to believe that protein should be avoided or minimized. We also do not get scurvy, yet diets that include a variety of plants rich in vitamin C are healthier than those that provide only the bare minimum. It seems that roughly 1 gram of protein per pound of lean body mass per day assures a good metabolic rate and high energy levels. Most find that they need a high-quality serving of protein with each meal to reach these levels. The meal plans provide for it.

Some of the recipes are complete meals, with protein, good carbs, and veggies already built in. Other recipes are just for healthy carbs or veggies. In those cases, include one of these protein options to make it complete.

**Sesame Orange Chicken** 134

**Baked Tofu** 137

**Almond Chicken Sauté** 138

**Baked Chicken** 139

**Baked Paprika Chicken with Brussels Sprouts** 140

**Creamy Shrimp and Tofu Soup** 142

**Lemon Baked Chicken** 143

**Baked Trout with Fennel** 144

**Poached Ginger Chicken** 146

**Poached Trout** 147

**Miso-Glazed Whitefish** 149

**Lime-Sautéed Scallops** 150

**Rosemary Citrus Chicken** 151

**Shredded Chicken** 152

**Trout en Papillote** 153

SYMPTOM KEY

- BF Brain fog
- F Fatigue
- HF Hot flashes
- I Insomnia
- W Weight gain

133

# Sesame Orange Chicken

**SERVES 4**
**Prep time:** 15 minutes
**Total time:** 30 minutes

SERVING SUGGESTION
Serve over rice as a complete meal.

RESET PHASE MODIFICATIONS
**ADRENAL RESET**
**Meal:** Lunch, dinner
**Modification:** Serve with rice as a complete meal.

**METABOLISM RESET**
**Meal:** Dinner
**Modification:** Serve with rice as a complete meal.

**THYROID RESET**
**Meal:** Any
**Modification:** None

GLUTEN-FREE OPTION
No modification needed

VEGAN OPTION
Use prepared seitan, cut into bite-size pieces, in place of chicken.

We don't eat out often, but one of my son's favorite meals is orange chicken. I worked hard to find a healthy version that he liked better than the one in restaurants, but it was worth it. Go slow when you toast the sesame seeds. As soon as you start to smell their flavor, they are about done. Once you have some rice ready, this recipe goes quickly. Start with the sauce, sauté the chicken, add veggies, garnish, and you're good to go!

Juice of 3 oranges (roughly 1½ cups)

¼ cup orange zest, freshly grated

1 tablespoon honey

2 garlic cloves, minced

1 tablespoon peeled and grated fresh ginger (about a 1-inch piece)

½ teaspoon crushed red pepper flakes

¼ cup tamari soy sauce

2 tablespoons apple cider vinegar

2 tablespoons raw white sesame seeds

2 tablespoons cornstarch or arrowroot flour

Misting oil

½ cup plus 2 tablespoons water, divided

2 chicken breasts, diced (about 1 pound)

2 cups broccoli florets

1 bunch scallions, washed, trimmed, sliced lengthwise into quarters, then cut into 1- to 2-inch pieces

Cooked brown rice for serving

Optional: Sriracha or other hot sauce for those who want more of a kick

- In a small saucepan, combine the orange juice, zest, honey, garlic, ginger, red pepper flakes, tamari, and vinegar. Bring to a light boil and simmer for 5 minutes.

- While the sauce is simmering, place a small skillet over medium-low heat and add the sesame seeds. Stirring often, dry-toast the sesame seeds for 2 to 3 minutes, or until lightly tanned and fragrant. Remove from the heat.

- In a small bowl, whisk the cornstarch into ½ cup of the water. Add to the sauce, simmer for a final 5 minutes, and remove from the heat.

- Mist the oil into a 12-inch skillet. Heat on medium-high until a drop of water sizzles. Put the chicken in the skillet, searing and stirring until just cooked, 5 to 7 minutes.

- Remove the chicken and set aside, keeping the drippings in the skillet.

- Sauté the broccoli with the remaining 2 tablespoons water in the skillet for 2 to 3 minutes, until it becomes brighter in color. Add the chicken and the sauce to the skillet. Simmer together for 2 to 3 minutes.

- Remove from the heat, spoon over the brown rice, garnish with the scallions and sesame seeds, and serve, adding sriracha to taste (if using).

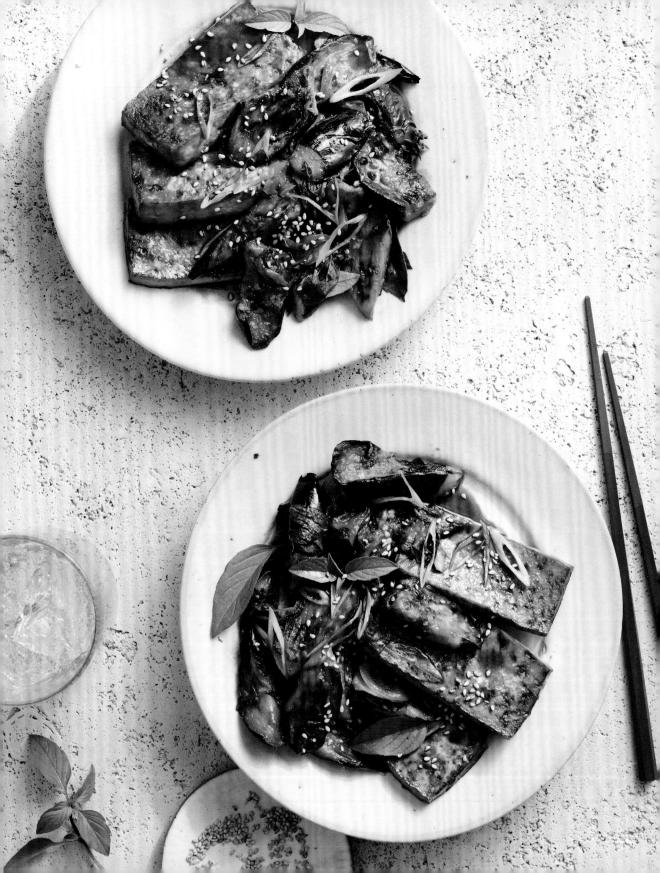

# Baked Tofu

SYMPTOMS IT CAN HELP

**HF** Hot flashes

**I** Insomnia

**SERVES 8**
**Prep time:** 20 minutes
**Total time:** 40 minutes

**RESET PHASE MODIFICATIONS**
**ADRENAL RESET**
**Meal:** Any
**Modification:** Serve with rice or another source of good carbs.

**METABOLISM RESET**
**Meal:** Dinner
**Modification:** Serve with rice or another source of good carbs.

**THYROID RESET**
**Meal:** Any
**Modification:** None

Nearly everyone loves tofu when it is seasoned and cooked well. You can find seasoned dried tofu in the stores, but it is easy to make your own. This is a good staple dish for batch-cooked protein.

2 blocks organic extra-firm tofu (12 to 15 ounces each)

2½ tablespoons tamari

1 teaspoon toasted sesame oil

1 tablespoon garlic salt

- Preheat the oven to 400°F.

- Cut the tofu into slices, each about ½ inch thick. Place a heavy towel on the counter and lay the slices on half of the towel. Fold the towel over the tofu so it is covered. Place a weight on the tofu. A cutting board with a heavy pan on top will serve. Press for 10 minutes.

- Place the pressed tofu in a bowl with the tamari, oil, and garlic salt. Mix well until the tofu is coated.

- Cover a baking sheet with parchment paper or a silicone mat. Arrange the tofu on the baking sheet with at least ½ inch of space between slices.

- Bake for 25 minutes and remove from the oven. Serve immediately or refrigerate for up to 5 days.

# Almond Chicken Sauté

SYMPTOMS IT CAN HELP

**BF** Brain fog

**F** Fatigue

**I** Insomnia

SERVES 4
**Prep time:** 10 minutes
**Total time:** 30 minutes

SERVING SUGGESTION
Serve over rice for a
complete meal.

RESET PHASE
MODIFICATIONS
**ADRENAL RESET**
**Meal:** Any
**Modification:** Serve with
rice or another source of
good carbs.

**METABOLISM RESET**
**Meal:** Dinner
**Modification:** Serve with
rice or another source of
good carbs.

**THYROID RESET**
**Meal:** Any
**Modification:** None

GLUTEN-FREE OPTION
Use gluten-free soy sauce.

VEGAN OPTIONS
Omit chicken or substitute
seitan or tempeh. Use
vegetable broth instead
of chicken broth.

Here is my version of the classic takeout dish. It is worth toasting the almonds, but there is a narrow window of opportunity between well-toasted and burnt. Sliced almonds are best, but chopped work, too.

½ cup sliced almonds

Misting oil

1 medium onion, peeled and diced

1 cup white button mushrooms, cleaned, stems removed, and sliced

1 zucchini, quartered lengthwise and sliced

2 boneless, skinless chicken breasts, diced into equal-size pieces

Kosher salt and freshly ground black pepper to taste

2 garlic cloves, minced

1 tablespoon peeled and minced fresh ginger

½ cup chicken broth

1 tablespoon soy sauce

1 teaspoon toasted sesame seed oil

1 teaspoon Sucanat or natural sweetener of choice

2 teaspoons cornstarch or arrowroot powder

- Heat the almonds in a sauté pan over low heat. Sauté, stirring frequently, until lightly toasted and fragrant, 1 to 2 minutes.

- Remove the almonds from the pan, add a fine mist of the oil, and raise the heat to medium-high. Add the onion and cook for 3 minutes, or until softened. Add the mushrooms and the zucchini and sauté an additional 3 minutes. Remove the vegetables and add another fine mist of oil.

- Add the chicken to the pan and lightly season with salt and pepper. Cook for 3 to 4 minutes, until cooked through; work in batches if needed so you don't crowd the pan. Add the garlic and the ginger, then sauté an extra minute.

- In a small bowl, combine the chicken broth, soy sauce, sesame oil, Sucanat, and cornstarch, mixing well.

- Add the sauce and the vegetables back to the pan. Sauté for 2 minutes, or until the sauce has thickened. Serve immediately over steamed rice.

# Baked Chicken

SYMPTOMS IT CAN HELP

**F** Fatigue

**W** Weight gain

**SERVES 8**
**Prep time:** 20 minutes
**Total time:** 35 minutes

RESET PHASE
MODIFICATIONS
**ADRENAL RESET**
**Meal:** Any
**Modification:** Serve with rice or another source of good carbs.

**METABOLISM RESET**
**Meal:** Dinner
**Modification:** Serve with rice or another source of good carbs.

**THYROID RESET**
**Meal:** Any
**Modification:** None

Family-size packs of chicken breasts are the best option for this recipe. Just make sure to watch the temperature so they do not come out overcooked. Chicken should be cooked to 165°F, but if you remove it from the oven at 160°F, it will continue to cook the rest of the way.

3 pounds boneless, skinless chicken breasts, trimmed of visible fat

1½ teaspoons kosher salt

■ Preheat the oven to 375°F.

■ Cut the chicken lengthwise into tenderloin strips about 1 inch in width.

■ Arrange the chicken on a baking sheet covered with parchment paper, leaving at least ½ inch of space between the pieces. Sprinkle salt on both sides of each strip.

■ Bake the chicken for 15 minutes and turn over. Bake an additional 10 minutes. Remove from the oven when the center reaches 160°F on a meat thermometer. Let cool for 5 minutes. Serve or refrigerate for up to 5 days.

# Baked Paprika Chicken with Brussels Sprouts

## SYMPTOMS IT CAN HELP

BF Brain fog

HF Hot flashes

I Insomnia

**SERVES 4**
**Prep time:** 20 minutes
**Total time:** 1 hour

**SERVING SUGGESTION**
Serve with rice or potatoes as a complete meal.

**RESET PHASE MODIFICATIONS**
**ADRENAL RESET**
**Meal:** Any
**Modification:** None

**METABOLISM RESET**
**Meal:** Dinner
**Modification:** Serve with carbs and without additional fat.

**THYROID RESET**
**Meal:** Any
**Modification:** None

**GLUTEN-FREE OPTION**
No modification needed

**VEGAN OPTION**
Omit chicken and replace with 1 pound of firm tofu, pressed.

Consider this one of the best go-to dishes for chicken. You can try it with most any vegetable combination, but Brussels sprouts are an excellent fit.

**SPICE BLEND**

1 tablespoon paprika

1 teaspoon Italian seasoning

1 teaspoon garlic powder

1 teaspoon onion powder

2 teaspoons kosher salt

Several grinds fresh black pepper

2 bone-in, skinless chicken breasts, split and pounded to a uniform thickness of roughly 1 inch

1 pound Brussels sprouts, trimmed and cut in half lengthwise

Misting oil

- Preheat the oven to 400°F.

- In a mixing bowl, whisk together the spice blend.

- Coat the chicken breasts on both sides with the spice blend. Place the chicken on a baking sheet covered with parchment paper, surrounded by the Brussels sprouts. Spray the chicken and sprouts with a fine mist of oil.

- Roast on the middle rack of the oven for 45 minutes, or until the sprouts are tender and the chicken has an internal temperature of at least 160°F on a meat thermometer.

- Let rest for 5 minutes and serve.

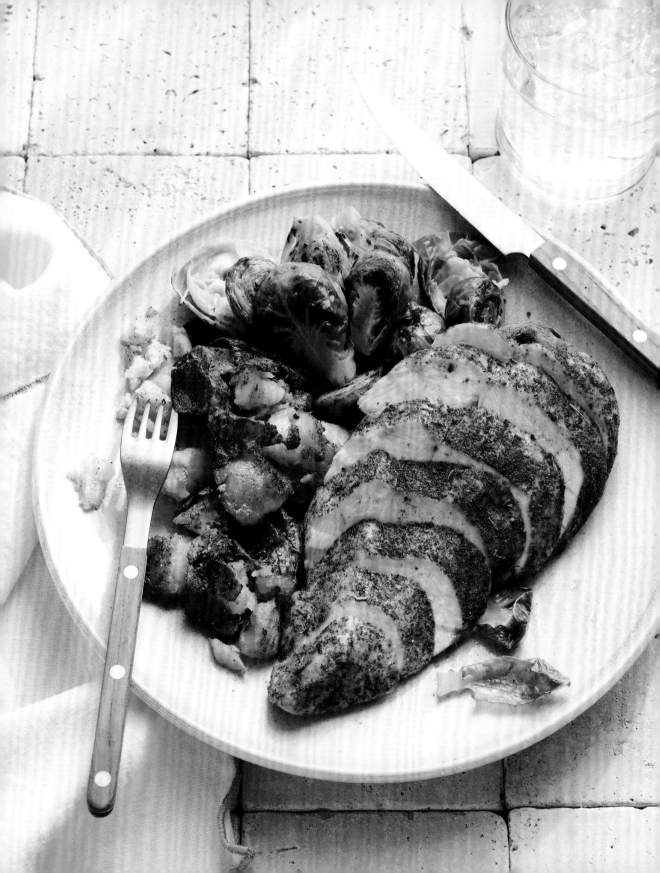

# Creamy Shrimp and Tofu Soup

In the United States, you rarely see tofu outside of vegetarian dishes. That is not the case in most of Asia. The taste and texture of tofu is a helpful addition to plenty of nonvegetarian dishes like this one. If you can't find Thai chili paste, you can use 1 tablespoon of chili powder.

8 ounces soft tofu

4 cups chicken broth, divided

Misting oil

6 cloves garlic, minced

1 tablespoon red Thai chili paste

½ cup tomato sauce

1 pound shrimp, peeled and deveined

1 medium carrot, sliced

¼ cup chopped cilantro

- In the bowl of a blender, combine the tofu with 1 cup of the broth until smooth.

- Mist a large pot with the oil and heat over medium heat. Add the garlic and cook 2 minutes, or until lightly browned. Add the chili paste and cook for an additional minute.

- Mix in the tomato sauce evenly. Stir in the tofu and the remaining broth. Simmer for 10 minutes, stirring occasionally.

- Add the shrimp and the carrot slices, and simmer for 3 to 4 minutes, or until shrimp is just cooked. Remove from heat, garnish with the cilantro, and serve.

# Lemon Baked Chicken

SYMPTOMS IT CAN HELP

**HF** Hot flashes

**I** Insomnia

**W** Weight gain

SERVES 4
**Prep time:** 5 minutes
**Total time:** 30 minutes

SERVING SUGGESTION
Serve with a healthy carb.

RESET PHASE
MODIFICATIONS
**ADRENAL RESET**
**Meal:** Lunch, dinner
**Modification:** Serve with
rice and veggies as a
complete meal.

**METABOLISM RESET**
**Meal:** Dinner
**Modification:** Serve with
rice and veggies as a
complete meal.

**THYROID RESET**
**Meal:** Any
**Modification:** None

GLUTEN-FREE OPTION
No modification needed

VEGAN OPTION
Use firm tofu in place of
chicken and vegetable
broth in place of chicken
broth.

Here is another good way to get your citrus. If you like planning ahead, feel free to use the liquid ingredients to marinate the chicken for anywhere from 30 to 60 minutes before baking it. You can also add some vegetables to one side of a lightly oiled baking sheet to roast them. Carrots, zucchini, cauliflower, and beets can cook for as long as the chicken. I like to pound out chicken breasts so that they have an even thickness. This way they are done at the same time, and none end up overcooked.

Misting oil

2 boneless, skinless chicken breasts, pounded out to a uniform thickness of 1 inch

1 small head cauliflower, cut into small florets

4 tablespoons fresh lemon juice (from approximately 2 lemons; slice lemons after juicing and save for garnish)

½ cup chicken broth

1 tablespoon honey

3 garlic cloves, minced

1 tablespoon dried oregano

1 teaspoon kosher salt or to taste

- Preheat the oven to 400°F. Lightly mist oil on a large sheet pan.

- Mist oil in a large skillet and heat on medium-high. Add the chicken and cook 2 to 3 minutes on each side until just browned. Remove the chicken from the pan and place on the baking sheet with the cauliflower and the lemon slices.

- In a small bowl, whisk together the chicken broth, lemon juice, honey, garlic, oregano, and salt.

- Pour the sauce over the chicken. Bake 20 to 30 minutes, ladling the sauce over the chicken every 5 minutes. Bake until the chicken is cooked through and reaches 160°F on a meat thermometer.

# Baked Trout with Fennel

SYMPTOMS IT CAN HELP

BF Brain fog

F Fatigue

I Insomnia

SERVES 4
**Prep time:** 15 minutes
**Total time:** 30 minutes

SERVING SUGGESTION
Serve with basmati rice or potatoes for a complete meal.

GLUTEN-FREE OPTION
No modification needed

VEGAN OPTION
Omit trout and replace with 1 pound of firm tofu, pressed.

This is one of those easy dishes that is sure to impress your audience. You'll want to serve the wrapped pouches right on the plate and let your guests open them up themselves.

4 trout fillets
(5 to 6 ounces each)

1 cup green peas, fresh or frozen and thawed

Zest and juice from 1 lemon

1 fennel bulb, finely sliced

1 teaspoon kosher salt

½ teaspoon white pepper

1 avocado, peeled, pitted, and cubed

- Preheat the oven to 350°F and cover a baking sheet with parchment paper.

- Place the trout, peas, lemon zest, and fennel in the center of the parchment paper and sprinkle with the salt and the pepper. Fold the ends of the parchment paper up to form a pouch and turn it over so that the weight of the food holds the pouch closed.

- Bake in the oven for 12 minutes. Open the package to check if the fish is soft and flaky. Return to the oven a few additional minutes, if needed.

- Remove from the oven and place on a serving plate, separating the fish from the vegetables. Stir the avocado into the vegetables and pour the lemon juice over the fish.

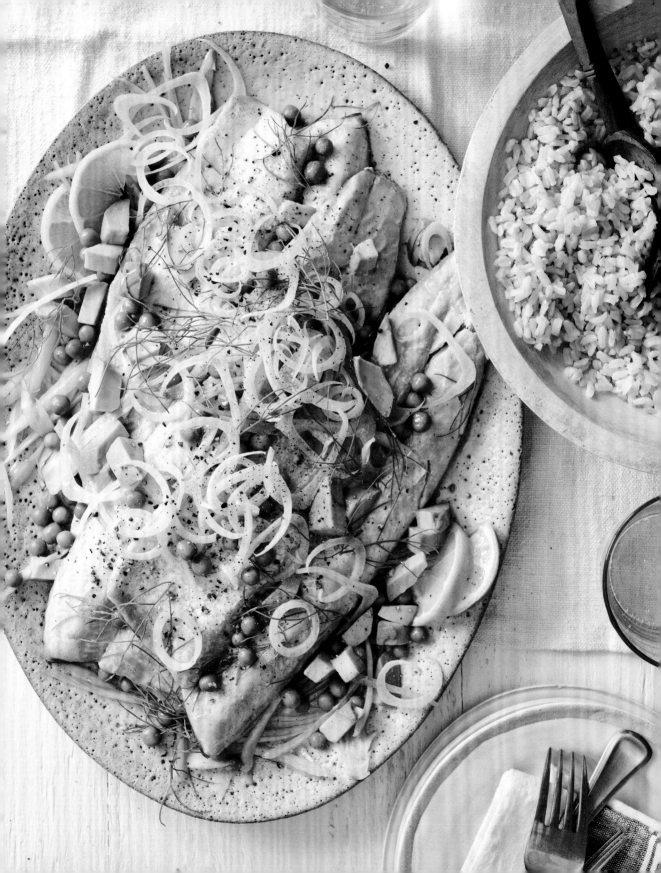

# Poached Ginger Chicken

SYMPTOMS IT CAN HELP

**F** Fatigue

**I** Insomnia

**W** Weight gain

SERVES 4
**Prep time:** 5 minutes
**Total time:** 15 minutes

SERVING SUGGESTION
Serve with greens or
a salad for a complete
meal.

RESET PHASE
MODIFICATIONS
**ADRENAL RESET**
**Meal:** Any
**Modification:** None

**METABOLISM RESET**
**Meal:** Dinner
**Modification:** Serve with
veggies.

**THYROID RESET**
**Meal:** Any
**Modification:** None

GLUTEN-FREE OPTION
No modification needed

VEGAN OPTION
Use firm tofu in place of
the chicken.

This is always one of my family's favorite quick meals when we have chicken and leftover rice. Basically, you are using massive amounts of garlic and ginger to flavor the broth, and the broth flavors the chicken. This is also a good vegan dish with tofu!

4 cups water

2 heads garlic, cut in half lengthwise

1 piece fresh ginger, 4 inches long, quartered

4 scallions, cleaned and ends trimmed

1 bunch cilantro, washed

2 jalapeños with tops, stems, and seeds removed, sliced into matchsticks

Juice of 1 lime

2 skinless boneless chicken breasts, each cut into 4 pieces

1 tablespoon kosher salt or to taste

2 cups cooked rice

- In a medium saucepan, bring the water to a boil, then reduce to a simmer.

- Add all the remaining ingredients except the rice and simmer until the chicken reaches 155°F on a meat thermometer. Strain out all the ingredients from the broth, adding the chicken and 2 of the scallions back in.

- Stir in the cooked rice and serve.

# Poached Trout

BF Brain fog

HF Hot flashes

I Insomnia

**SERVES 8**
**Prep time:** 5 minutes
**Total time:** 15 minutes

SERVING SUGGESTION
Serve with vegetables
and good carbs of your
choice for a quick meal.

RESET PHASE
MODIFICATIONS
**ADRENAL RESET**
**Meal:** Lunch, dinner
**Modification:** Serve with
rice and veggies as a
complete meal.

**METABOLISM RESET**
**Meal:** Dinner
**Modification:** Serve with
rice and veggies as a
complete meal.

**THYROID RESET**
**Meal:** Any
**Modification:** None

GLUTEN-FREE OPTION
No modification needed

VEGAN OPTION
Use tempeh instead of
trout.

Here is a way to batch-cook fish for future recipes. Cooking times will vary based on the thickness of the fillets, so be sure to measure the temperature. One key trick to precooking fish is to intentionally undercook it, just a bit. If you plan on serving it right away, cook all the way to 135°F and let sit for five minutes before serving.

3 quarts water

3 tablespoons
kosher salt

1 or 2 large trout
fillets, roughly 1½ to
2½ pounds total
weight, cut into
8 (4- to 6-ounce)
servings

- In a 6-quart stockpot, bring the water to a boil and add the salt. Using a slotted spoon, lower the fish into the water.

- Cook for roughly 5 to 7 minutes, or until the internal temperature of the fish reaches 135°F on a meat thermometer. Scoop the fish out of the water and let it cool for 20 minutes before refrigerating.

- Wrap the fish in a layer of parchment paper and place inside an airtight storage container. Refrigerate for up to 5 days.

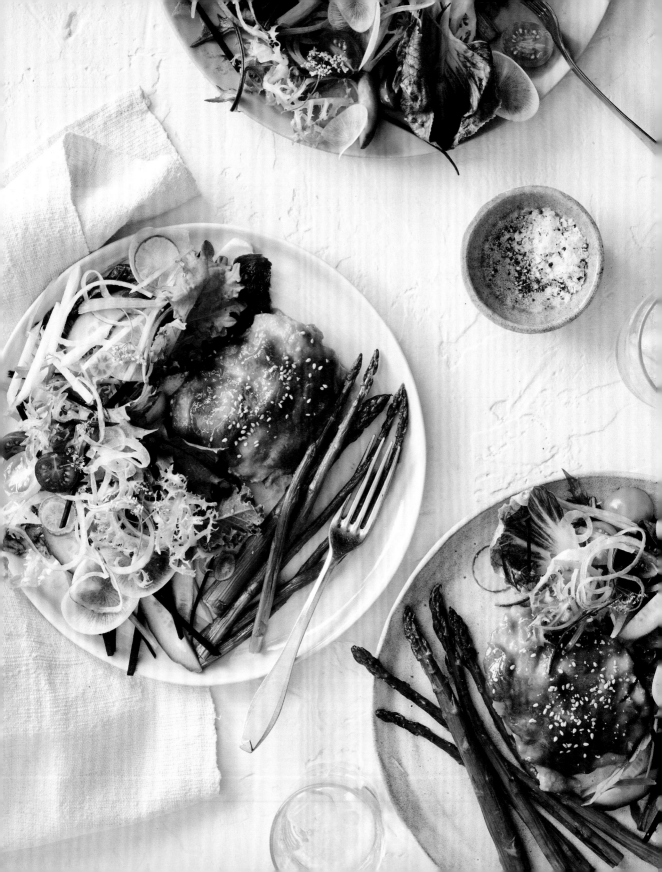

# Miso-Glazed Whitefish

## SYMPTOMS IT CAN HELP

**BF** Brain fog

**I** Insomnia

**W** Weight gain

## SERVES 4
**Prep time:** 10 minutes
**Total time:** 25 minutes

## SERVING SUGGESTION
Serve immediately along with rice for a complete meal.

## RESET PHASE MODIFICATIONS
**ADRENAL RESET**
**Meal:** Lunch, dinner
**Modification:** Serve with rice as a complete meal.

**METABOLISM RESET**
**Meal:** Dinner
**Modification:** Serve with rice as a complete meal.

**THYROID RESET**
**Meal:** Any
**Modification:** None

## GLUTEN-FREE OPTION
No modification needed

## VEGAN OPTION
Omit fish and replace with 1½ pounds of extra-firm tofu.

Look for a white miso paste for this recipe. You can find it in the refrigerated section of larger grocery stores. I use rockfish, but any whitefish or salmon can work. Be sure to choose a low-iodine fish if you're on the Thyroid Reset Diet.

5 tablespoons white miso paste

2 tablespoons mirin

1½ tablespoons honey

2 tablespoons tamari soy sauce

1 (1-inch) piece fresh ginger, peeled and minced

4 (6- to 8-ounce) rockfish fillets

1 bunch asparagus, trimmed

Kosher salt and freshly ground black pepper

- Preheat the oven to 450°F.

- In a medium bowl, combine the miso, mirin, honey, tamari, and ginger. Stir into a paste. Coat both sides of the fillets with the paste and let them marinate for 10 minutes.

- Place the asparagus on a baking sheet in four groups. Place 1 piece of the fish over each group of asparagus. Add salt and pepper to taste.

- Place the baking sheet in the oven for 15 minutes, or until the fish starts to flake.

# Lime-Sautéed Scallops

SYMPTOMS IT CAN HELP

F Fatigue

HF Hot flashes

I Insomnia

**SERVES 4**
**Prep time:** 5 minutes
**Total time:** 15 minutes

SERVING SUGGESTION
Serve with leftover bread, rice, or noodles and a salad.

RESET PHASE MODIFICATIONS
**ADRENAL RESET**
**Meal:** Lunch, dinner
**Modification:** Serve with rice as a complete meal.

**METABOLISM RESET**
**Meal:** Dinner
**Modification:** Serve with rice as a complete meal.

**THYROID RESET**
**Meal:** Any
**Modification:** None

GLUTEN-FREE OPTION
No modification needed

VEGAN OPTION
Substitute tofu. Rinse and slice firm tofu into rectangles ½ to ¾ inch thick. Place slices between layers of a dish towel and place a weight on top. Press for 20 or more minutes, then use in place of scallops.

Scallops are not a common choice, but they are one of the best low-iodine seafood options. This is an easy and impressive dish. The two tricks that make this recipe shine are to get fresh scallops and to sear them quickly. If you can't find fresh scallops, you can use frozen instead. They should need only an hour or so to thaw if you place them on a metal baking sheet at room temperature, turning them over halfway through.

1 pound sea scallops

2 teaspoons kosher salt

Misting oil

Freshly ground black pepper to taste

2 tablespoons chopped cilantro

1 garlic clove, minced

2 teaspoons fresh lime juice

- Rinse and pat dry each scallop. Sprinkle with the salt.

- Mist the oil into a 12-inch or larger skillet with a cover. Heat on medium-high until a drop of water sizzles. Place the scallops in the pan, spaced at least ½ inch apart. Let the scallops sear for 1 minute.

- Turn the scallops over one at a time and sprinkle with the pepper after turning. Sear 1 minute longer. When you finish, add the cilantro, garlic, and lime juice to the pan. Cover and let steam for 1 minute.

- Remove from the heat and serve immediately.

# Rosemary Citrus Chicken

SYMPTOMS IT CAN HELP

BF Brain fog

HF Hot flashes

I Insomnia

**SERVES 4**
**Prep time:** 10 minutes
**Total time:** 30 minutes

SERVING SUGGESTION
Serve over cooked rice.

RESET PHASE
MODIFICATIONS
**ADRENAL RESET**
**Meal:** Lunch, dinner
**Modification:** Serve with rice as a complete meal.

**METABOLISM RESET**
**Meal:** Dinner
**Modification:** Serve with rice as a complete meal.

**THYROID RESET**
**Meal:** Any
**Modification:** None

GLUTEN-FREE OPTION
No modification needed

VEGAN OPTION
Use tempeh instead of chicken and vegetable broth instead of chicken broth.

This is a simple light dish that makes a good staple for weeknights. If you are planning to serve with rice, you can stir in cooked rice for the final 15 minutes of baking.

2 boneless, skinless chicken breasts (about 1½ pounds)

Kosher salt and freshly ground black pepper to taste

Misting oil

2 teaspoons minced fresh rosemary leaves

2 cloves garlic, minced

¼ cup chicken broth

Juice of 1 lemon (about 3 tablespoons)

2 tablespoons chopped fresh parsley leaves

- Preheat the oven to 400°F and lightly oil a 9×13-inch baking dish.

- Sprinkle the chicken breasts on both sides with the salt and pepper. Mist oil into a large pan and heat on medium-high. Add the chicken breasts and cook for 3 to 5 minutes on each side, or until browned.

- Transfer the chicken to the oiled baking dish.

- In a small bowl, combine the rosemary, garlic, chicken broth, and lemon juice. Pour the mixture over the chicken. Bake for 25 minutes, or until the chicken reaches 165°F on a meat thermometer.

- Ladle the sauce from the bottom of the baking dish over the chicken, sprinkle with the parsley, and serve.

# Shredded Chicken

SYMPTOMS IT CAN HELP

**BF** Brain fog

**F** Fatigue

**HF** Hot flashes

**I** Insomnia

**W** Weight gain

SERVES 8
**Prep time:** 5 minutes
**Total time:** 2 hours

SERVING SUGGESTION
Serve with vegetables
and healthy carbs of your
choice for a quick meal.

RESET PHASE
MODIFICATIONS
**ADRENAL RESET**
**Meal:** Any
**Modification:** Serve with
rice or another source of
good carbs.

**METABOLISM RESET**
**Meal:** Dinner
**Modification:** Serve with
rice or another source of
good carbs.

**THYROID RESET**
**Meal:** Any
**Modification:** None

You'll be amazed at how easy and flavorful this one-ingredient dish is!
It is versatile enough to use as a source of protein with nearly any meal.
The trick is slow cooking at low temperature.

Avocado oil,
for misting

3 to 5 medium
chicken breasts
(roughly 1½ to
2½ pounds total
weight)

■ Mist the oil into a 2- to 3-quart saucepan with a tight-fitting lid. Heat
on medium-high until a drop of water sizzles.

■ Place the chicken breasts in the pot so that they cover as much of
the bottom as possible. Turn to the lowest simmer setting and let
cook for 1 hour and 45 minutes to 2 hours. Cooking times may vary
based on individual stove settings. The chicken is done when it
shreds with light pressure from a fork.

■ Remove from heat and use a large fork or a masher to break up
the chicken, mixing it in with the liquid that has formed. Place it in a
glass storage container with a tight-fitting lid, allowing the chicken
to cool for 30 minutes before refrigerating.

■ Use as a source of neutral-flavored protein in a range of recipes.
Refrigerate for up to 5 days.

# Trout en Papillote

SYMPTOMS IT CAN HELP

BF Brain fog

F Fatigue

W Weight gain

**SERVES 4**
**Prep time:** 10 minutes
**Total time:** 25 minutes

**SERVING SUGGESTION**
Serve immediately along with rice for a complete meal.

**RESET PHASE MODIFICATIONS**
**ADRENAL RESET**
**Meal:** Lunch, dinner
**Modification:** Serve with rice as a complete meal.

**METABOLISM RESET**
**Meal:** Dinner
**Modification:** Serve with rice as a complete meal.

**THYROID RESET**
**Meal:** Any
**Modification:** None

**GLUTEN-FREE OPTION**
No modification needed

**VEGAN OPTION**
Omit trout and replace with 1½ pounds of extra-firm tofu.

The French phrase *en papillote* just means "in paper," and it refers to the technique of baking a dish in a pouch. The pouch retains the moisture and blends the flavors of all the ingredients. You can use this method with other types of seafood or poultry. Normally I use parchment paper to create the pouch, but aluminum foil is another option.

1 medium onion, sliced thin

1 green bell pepper, cored, seeded, and cut into matchsticks

1½ pounds fresh trout

16 cherry tomatoes, halved

16 kalamata olives, halved

2 tablespoons capers

2 garlic cloves, minced

1 tablespoon lemon zest

2 teaspoons dried oregano

Kosher salt and freshly ground black pepper to taste

- Preheat the oven to 400°F.

- Tear four 12-inch sections of parchment paper and lay them out on the counter.

- Divide the onion and green pepper and place equal amounts in a rectangle on the center of each piece of parchment paper. Divide the trout into 4 equal-size servings and place one on top of each set of onion and green pepper. Divide the cherry tomatoes, olives, capers, garlic, lemon zest, and oregano and add them equally to the top of each piece of trout. Add the salt and pepper.

- Fold each piece over to make a sealed pouch, tucking the loose end of the paper underneath so that the weight holds it shut. Set all 4 pieces on a baking sheet and place in the oven for 15 minutes. Open the package and check for doneness. The trout is done when it starts to flake under gentle pressure.

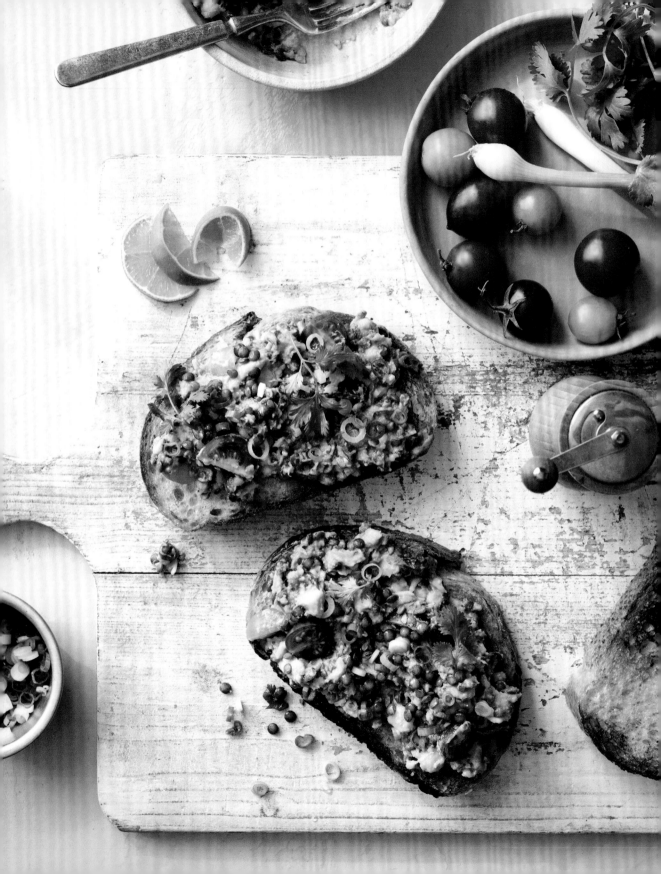

# Healthy Carbs

Carbohydrates are important elements of the diet because they are our primary fuel source and the only source of fibers to feed the microflora. Unprocessed carbohydrates have been the dietary staple of the world's healthiest cultures. The Mediterranean, traditional Asian, and Nordic diets are all centered around good carbs.

Here you'll find several healthy carb recipes to round out other meals. Carbs have the advantages of being cost-effective and easy to batch-cook, and they can be stored for many days after cooking.

SYMPTOM KEY

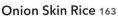

BF  Brain fog
F   Fatigue
HF  Hot flashes
I   Insomnia
W   Weight gain

# Lentil Avocado Smash

SYMPTOMS IT CAN HELP

**BF** Brain fog

**W** Weight gain

SERVES 4
**Prep time:** 5 minutes
**Total time:** 5 minutes

SERVING SUGGESTION
Serve as the base for a
sandwich or salad.

RESET PHASE
MODIFICATIONS
**ADRENAL RESET**
**Meal:** Any
**Modification:** None

**METABOLISM RESET**
**Meal:** Dinner
**Modification:** Serve as
base for salad with salad
veggies.

**THYROID RESET**
**Meal:** Any
**Modification:** None

GLUTEN-FREE OPTION
No modification needed

VEGAN OPTION
No modification needed

This is a healthier version of the classic avocado toast. Chickpeas can also be used in place of lentils. You do want to be sure the avocado is ripe so that it can be easily mashed.

1 cup cooked dried lentils or canned lentils, drained

2 medium avocados, peeled and pitted

8 cherry tomatoes, quartered

¼ cup chopped cilantro leaves

2 scallions, trimmed and sliced

Juice of 1 lime

½ teaspoon kosher salt

¼ teaspoon cayenne powder

■ Place all the ingredients into a medium bowl. Mash with a potato masher until the avocado is mostly broken up and all is well mixed.

■ Serve and enjoy.

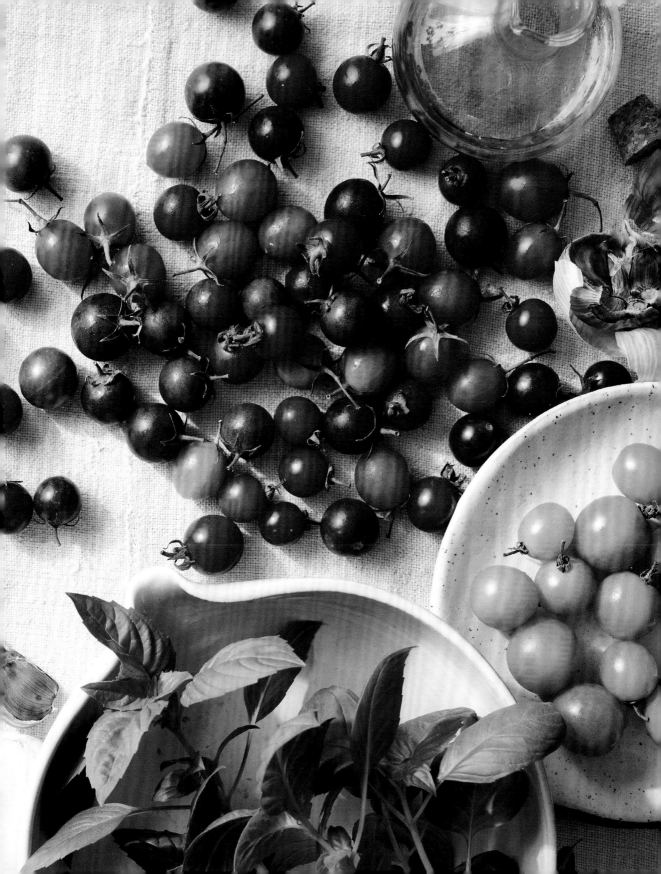

# Seasoned Lentils

## SYMPTOMS IT CAN HELP

**BF** Brain fog

**F** Fatigue

**HF** Hot flashes

**I** Insomnia

**W** Weight gain

**SERVES 4**
**Prep time:** 5 minutes
**Total time:** 25 minutes

**SERVING SUGGESTION**
Serve as a complete meal.

**RESET PHASE MODIFICATIONS**
**ADRENAL RESET**
**Meal:** Any
**Modification:** None

**METABOLISM RESET**
**Meal:** Dinner
**Modification:** None

**THYROID RESET**
**Meal:** Any
**Modification:** None

**GLUTEN-FREE OPTION**
No modification needed

**VEGAN OPTION**
No modification needed

Lentils are so good when they are well seasoned. They have such a perfect proportion of carbs and protein that a dish like this can make a complete meal. Just use plenty of cilantro or add some spinach to cover the bases for your veggies! You can use brown or red lentils. The only difference between them is that the red lentils have the outer skin removed, and so they cook a little faster.

1 cup dried brown or red lentils

3 cups vegetable broth

3 cups water

1 teaspoon olive oil

3 cloves garlic, minced

1 (8-ounce) can tomato sauce

1 tablespoon fresh lemon juice

½ teaspoon ground ginger

1 teaspoon ground cumin

½ teaspoon turmeric powder

1 teaspoon paprika

2 tablespoons chopped cilantro

- Add all the ingredients except the cilantro to a medium saucepan and bring to a simmer over medium heat.

- Simmer until the lentils are soft, watching and adding water if needed. Cook roughly 10 to 15 minutes for red lentils or 20 minutes for brown lentils.

- Serve topped with cilantro and enjoy!

# Caramelized Onion Pudding

SERVES 4
**Prep time:** 15 minutes
**Total time:** 1 hour and 5 minutes

SERVING SUGGESTION
Serve as a vegetable side dish.

RESET PHASE MODIFICATIONS
**ADRENAL RESET**
**Meal:** Any
**Modification:** None

**METABOLISM RESET**
**Meal:** Dinner
**Modification:** Serve in place of other carbs.

**THYROID RESET**
**Meal:** Any
**Modification:** None

GLUTEN-FREE OPTION
Use a gluten-free all-purpose flour like Bob's Red Mill.

VEGAN OPTION
Omit the egg whites and add ½ cup of flaxseed mixed into ½ cup of water.

Yes, onions by themselves work great as a side dish or as a dessert! This recipe lets you appreciate their natural sweetness. This dish starts out a lot like Lean French Onion Soup (page 185), but it ends up in the oven. If you can't find sweet onions, use yellow or white onions and add 1 teaspoon of Sucanat just before baking. For milk, I like to use unsweetened flax milk or skim milk. Any unflavored milk substitute can work well. It is just as good served cold the next day as it is right out of the oven.

| | | |
|---|---|---|
| 1 teaspoon neutral oil | ½ teaspoon water, if needed | ½ teaspoon kosher salt |
| 2 large sweet onions, thinly sliced | 1 tablespoon all-purpose flour | ½ cup unsweetened flax milk |
| | 4 egg whites | |

- Preheat the oven to 350°F. Lightly oil a 9-inch pie pan.

- Heat the oil in a large stockpot over medium heat until it starts to shimmer. Reduce the heat to medium-low and add the onions. Stir frequently and sauté for 20 to 30 minutes, or until lightly caramelized. Add the water if the onions start to stick.

- In a medium bowl, thoroughly mix the flour, egg whites, salt, and milk. Stir the cooked onions into the flour-and-egg mixture.

- Pour the batter into the lightly oiled pie pan. Bake for 40 minutes, or until lightly browned. Let rest 10 minutes before serving.

- Serve as a dessert or a vegetable side dish.

# Beet Cookies

## SYMPTOMS IT CAN HELP

**BF** Brain fog

**F** Fatigue

**I** Insomnia

**SERVES 8**
**Prep time:** 3 minutes
**Total time:** 15 minutes

**SERVING SUGGESTION**
Serve as dessert after a meal or as a snack.

**RESET PHASE MODIFICATIONS**
**ADRENAL RESET**
**Meal:** Lunch, dinner
**Modification:** Serve in place of other sources of carbs and fat.

**METABOLISM RESET**
**Meal:** Dinner
**Modification:** Serve in place of other sources of carbs and fat.

**THYROID RESET**
**Meal:** Any
**Modification:** None

**GLUTEN-FREE OPTION**
No modification needed

**VEGAN OPTION**
Omit the egg whites and add ¼ cup of flaxseed mixed into ¼ cup of water.

Both the taste and the color of these cookies are remarkable! Bring them to your next potluck and you'll be the star of the show. If you don't have any fresh beets on hand, canned beets work fine. Plus, they are easy to puree—you can just mash them with a fork.

¼ cup precooked or canned beets, pureed

½ cup almond butter

1 egg white

¼ cup Sucanat or natural sweetener of choice

1 tablespoon tapioca flour

1 teaspoon vanilla extract

Optional: ¼ cup carob or chocolate chips of your choice

- Preheat the oven to 375°F.

- Combine the beets, almond butter, egg white, and Sucanat in a medium bowl and mix thoroughly. Stir in the remaining ingredients.

- Form the batter into roughly 3-inch circles and flatten them. They will not spread, so you can space them as closely as 1 inch apart.

- Bake for 10 minutes or until an inserted toothpick comes out dry. Remove from the oven, let cool, and enjoy.

- Store for up to 3 days in an airtight container at room temperature.

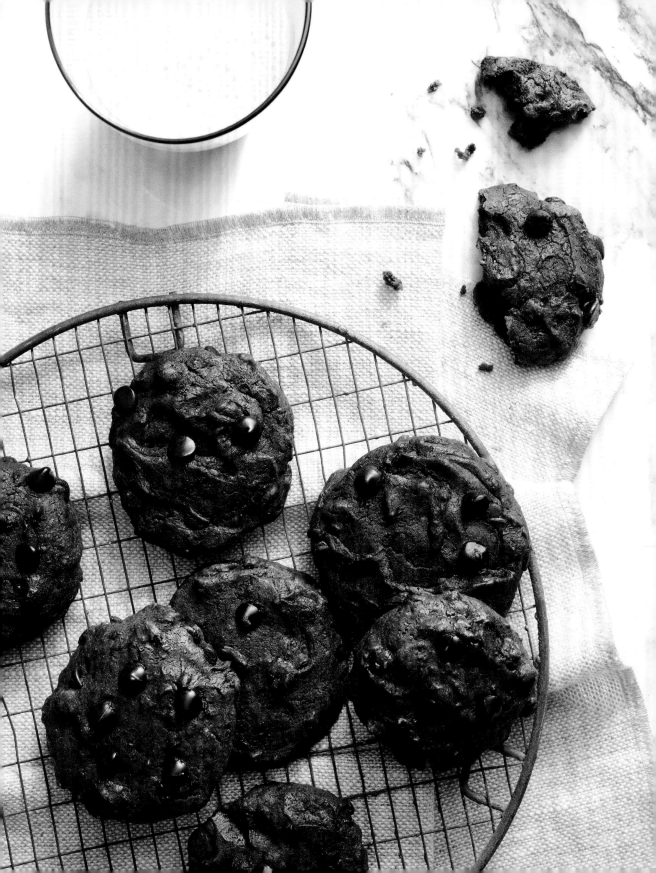

# Steel Cut Oat Risotto

## SYMPTOMS IT CAN HELP

BF Brain fog

F Fatigue

I Insomnia

## SERVES 4
**Prep time:** 5 minutes
**Total time:** 35 minutes

## SERVING SUGGESTION
Serve with a protein and vegetable dish for a quick meal.

## RESET PHASE MODIFICATIONS
**ADRENAL RESET**
**Meal:** Any
**Modification:** Serve in place of all other sources of carbs.

**METABOLISM RESET**
**Meal:** Dinner
**Modification:** Serve in place of all other sources of carbs.

**THYROID RESET**
**Meal:** Any
**Modification:** None

## GLUTEN-FREE OPTION
No modification needed

## VEGAN OPTION
Use vegetable bouillon in place of the chicken stock.

I've come to like the flavor of this savory oat dish better than traditional risottos. Of course, the oats also make it higher in phytonutrients and fibers.

Misting oil

1 leek, white and softer green parts, rinsed, quartered lengthwise, and finely sliced

1 cup steel cut oats

5 cups chicken stock

1 cup frozen peas

1 scallion, thinly sliced

¼ teaspoon ground white pepper

1 teaspoon kosher salt or to taste

- Coat a medium saucepan with a fine mist of oil. Heat over medium-high until the oil shimmers.

- Add the leeks and sauté until soft, 2 to 3 minutes. Add the oats and sauté for 2 minutes, or until fragrant. Add 1 cup of the stock and stir until absorbed. Repeat, adding 1 cup of the stock at a time and stirring it in until nearly absorbed before adding more.

- Once all the broth is incorporated, cook covered at a low simmer until the oats are tender, roughly 30 minutes. Stir in the peas and the scallion slices and continue to cook until both are heated through. Add the pepper and salt before serving.

# Onion Skin Rice

**SYMPTOMS IT CAN HELP**

BF Brain fog

W Weight gain

**SERVES 8**
**Prep time:** 5 minutes
**Total time:** 50 minutes

**SERVING SUGGESTION**
Serve as a source of carbs
for any meal.

**RESET PHASE**
**MODIFICATIONS**
**ADRENAL RESET**
**Meal:** Any
**Modification:** None

**METABOLISM RESET**
**Meal:** Dinner
**Modification:** Serve in
place of other carbs.

**THYROID RESET**
**Meal:** Any
**Modification:** None

**GLUTEN-FREE OPTION**
No modification needed

**VEGAN OPTION**
No modification needed

Onion skins are the densest dietary source of quercetin and related bioflavonoids. They can be saved for vegetable broth, or you can add them to your rice. You can even include the root hairs that are attached to the skin. Just pick the skins off the top after the cooking is done, because all of the phytonutrients transfer into the rice.

Misting oil

½ medium onion, diced

1 garlic clove, minced

2 cups brown basmati rice, rinsed

1½ cups water

1 teaspoon fresh turmeric powder

2 cups vegetable broth

1 bay leaf

½ teaspoon kosher salt

Skins from 1 to 3 onions

- Mist a medium saucepan with the oil. Heat on medium-high until the oil shimmers. Sauté the onion and garlic for 2 minutes, or until soft.

- Add the rice and sauté an additional 2 to 3 minutes, or until fragrant. Add all the remaining ingredients.

- Simmer on low for 35 minutes, turn off the heat, and let sit, covered, for 10 minutes. Remove the onion skins from the top and serve.

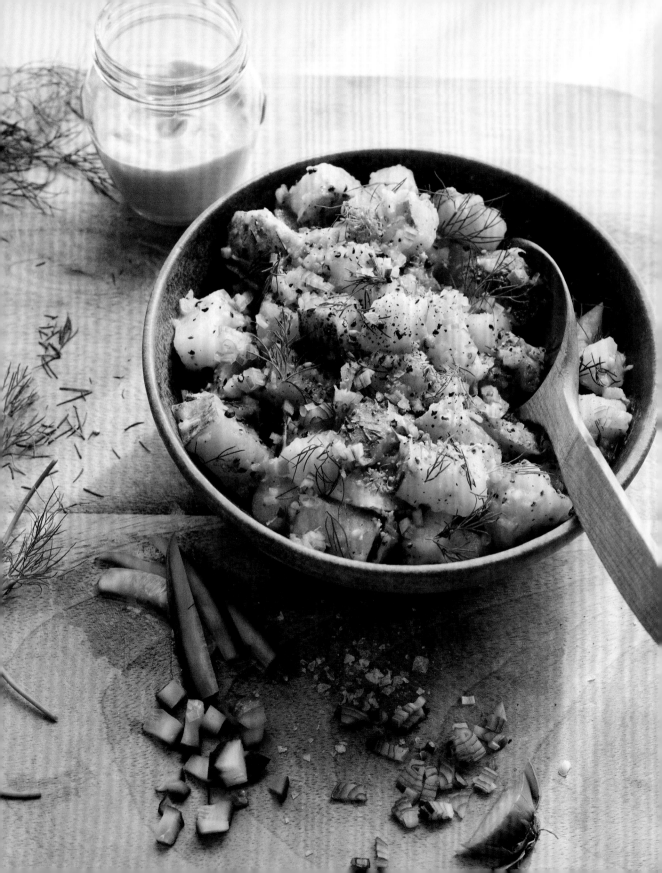

# Dr. C's Potato Salad

SYMPTOMS IT CAN HELP

BF Brain fog

F Fatigue

W Weight gain

**SERVES 4**
**Prep time:** 5 minutes
**Total time:** 25 minutes

**SERVING SUGGESTION**
Serve with a source
of protein and other
optional veggies for a
complete meal.

**RESET PHASE
MODIFICATIONS**
**ADRENAL RESET**
**Meal:** Any
**Modification:** None

**METABOLISM RESET**
**Meal:** Dinner
**Modification:** Serve in
place of other carbs.

**THYROID RESET**
**Meal:** Any
**Modification:** None

**GLUTEN-FREE OPTION**
No modification needed

**VEGAN OPTION**
No modification needed

I love potato salads, but most use way too much mayonnaise. Fresh dill is a wonderful addition. Russets work the best for this salad, but any potatoes are worth using, especially if you have leftovers. You can also use ⅓ cup finely diced red onion in place of the shallots.

2 pounds russet
potatoes, washed
and cut into 1-inch
cubes

2 tablespoons
kosher salt

**DRESSING**

½ tablespoon
olive oil

2 tablespoons
fresh lemon juice

2 teaspoons
Dijon mustard

2 medium shallots,
finely diced

2 teaspoons finely
chopped fresh dill

¼ cup pickle relish
or diced pickles

Kosher salt and
freshly ground black
pepper to taste

- Place the potatoes in a large pot. Cover with water and stir in the salt. Bring to a boil and cook for 8 minutes or until the potatoes are fork-tender. Drain and rinse the potatoes under cold water.

- Whisk the dressing ingredients together in a serving bowl until well blended. Stir the potatoes into the bowl with the dressing and serve.

# Rosemary Roasted Potatoes

## SYMPTOMS IT CAN HELP

 Brain fog

Hot flashes

Insomnia

**SERVES 4**
**Prep time:** 10 minutes
**Total time:** 40 minutes

**SERVING SUGGESTION**
Serve as a side dish of
healthy carbs.

**RESET PHASE
MODIFICATIONS**
**ADRENAL RESET**
**Meal:** Any
**Modification:** Serve in
place of other carbs.

**METABOLISM RESET**
**Meal:** Dinner
**Modification:** Serve in
place of other carbs.

**THYROID RESET**
**Meal:** Any
**Modification:** None

**GLUTEN-FREE OPTION**
No modification needed

**VEGAN OPTION**
Use tempeh instead
of chicken and vegetable
broth instead of
chicken broth.

Yep, another potato dish. You may have heard me talk about how boiled potatoes contain resistant starch. Roasted potatoes are also rich in resistant starch, just not as much as boiled. You can roast these and refrigerate them overnight before serving for more-resistant starch. Nonetheless, they are still good options for variety. In this recipe, consider them an excellent vehicle to provide the benefits of rosemary. Red potatoes are best for roasting. Based on their size, quartering usually works. You want to end up with wedges that are 1½ to 2½ inches long.

Misting oil

2 pounds red
potatoes, peeled
and quartered

Juice of ½ lemon

1 teaspoon
kosher salt

Freshly ground
black pepper
to taste

2 tablespoons
chopped fresh
rosemary

- Preheat the oven to 450°F.

- Lightly mist the potatoes with the oil. In a medium bowl, stir together the potatoes, lemon juice, salt, and pepper.

- Spread the potatoes on a baking pan lightly misted with oil. Roast for 30 minutes, stirring the potatoes every 10 minutes. Add the rosemary to the potatoes and stir thoroughly and evenly.

- Roast a final 10 minutes and serve.

# Garlic Mashed Potatoes

## SYMPTOMS IT CAN HELP

**BF** Brain fog

**F** Fatigue

**HF** Hot flashes

**SERVES 4**
**Prep time:** 5 minutes
**Total time:** 30 minutes

**SERVING SUGGESTION**
Use as a side dish for lunch or dinner.

**RESET PHASE MODIFICATIONS**

**ADRENAL RESET**
**Meal:** Any
**Modification:** Serve in place of other sources of carbs.

**METABOLISM RESET**
**Meal:** Dinner
**Modification:** Serve in place of other sources of carbs.

**THYROID RESET**
**Meal:** Any
**Modification:** None

**GLUTEN-FREE OPTION**
No modification needed

**VEGAN OPTION**
No modification needed

Pair this with any savory dish, but don't add gravy, because the flavor of the potatoes is too bold. Next time you roast garlic, roast several heads at a time. You can use russet or red potatoes, but the flavor of Yukon Golds works best.

| | | |
|---|---|---|
| 2 pounds Yukon Gold potatoes, peeled and quartered | 3 tablespoons kosher salt, plus 1 teaspoon | 1 teaspoon snipped fresh chives for garnish |
| | 2 roasted bulbs garlic (see page 219), skins removed | |

- Place the potatoes in a large pot and cover with cold water by 1 inch and 3 tablespoons of the salt.

- Bring to a boil and cook for 10 to 12 minutes, or until the potatoes are easily split with a fork. Drain the potatoes, reserving 1 cup of the starchy cooking water.

- Using a fork, mash the garlic into a puree. Add the garlic, the reserved cooking water, the remaining teaspoon salt, and the potatoes to a medium bowl. Use a masher to blend everything evenly.

- Garnish with the chives and serve.

# Crispy Mashed Potatoes

I've never met a potato I didn't like! These take a bit more time, but you might find they are worth it. This recipe works best with small potatoes–new potatoes or baby potatoes. If you want to get wild, try making this dish with smaller purple- or red-fleshed potatoes.

14 red potatoes

2 tablespoons
kosher salt

Misting oil

1 teaspoon
garlic powder

1 teaspoon paprika

Kosher salt and
freshly ground black
pepper to taste

- Preheat the oven to 425°F.

- Place the potatoes in a large pot. Cover with water and stir in the salt. Bring to a boil and cook for 10 minutes, or until the potatoes are fork-tender.

- Drain and rinse the potatoes under cold water. Place each potato on a baking sheet and lightly smash it with a small bowl. Mist the potatoes with the oil and sprinkle with the garlic powder, paprika, salt, and pepper.

- Roast for 20 to 30 minutes, until golden brown.

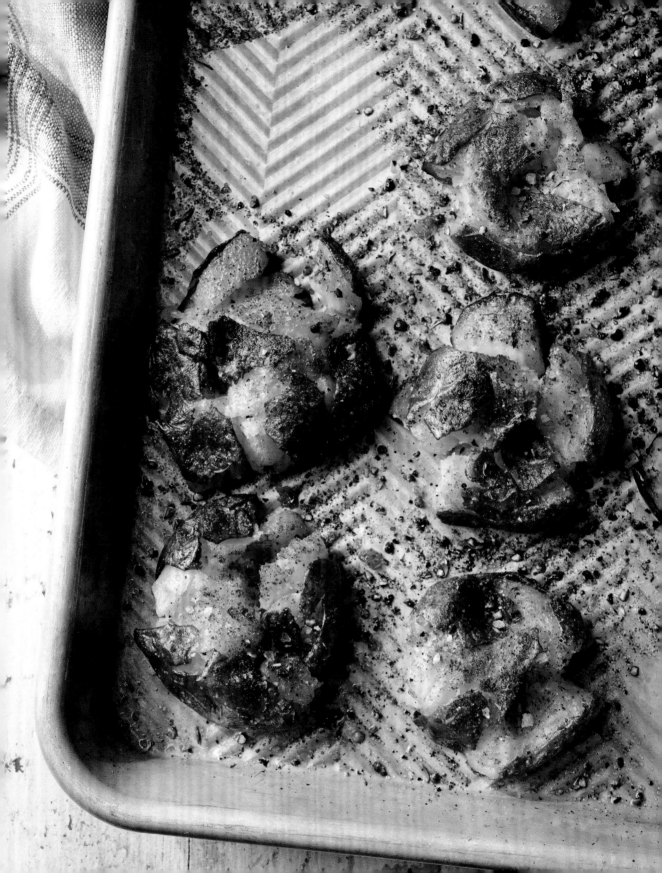

# Artisan Bread

SYMPTOMS IT CAN HELP

**BF** Brain fog

**F** Fatigue

**W** Weight gain

SERVES 8
**Prep time:** 5 minutes
**Total time:** 45 minutes + rising time

SERVING SUGGESTION
Serve as a side dish of healthy carbs.

GLUTEN-FREE OPTION
Use 3 cups gluten-free baking flour and omit the bread flour and whole wheat flour. Use ¼ cup gluten-free flour for loosening the dough from the bowl.

VEGAN OPTION
No modification needed

Here is our family's staple bread recipe. If you wish to have the benefits of sourdough, let it rise for 24 to 36 hours. The naturally occurring bacteria in the air will aid in the process.

2½ cups bread flour, plus ¼ cup more for loosening the dough from bowl

½ cup whole wheat flour

1 tablespoon kosher salt

1½ cups warm water

1 teaspoon yeast

- Mix all the ingredients (except the additional ¼ cup bread flour) in a large steel or glass prep bowl and stir a few dozen times. The dough will be between the texture of batter and typical bread dough. It will not all stay together. It does not require thorough mixing or kneading.

- Cover with a damp towel and let rise in a warm place for 2 to 36 hours. If you prefer more of a sourdough flavor, let it sit for 24 to 36 hours.

- Place a 4-quart Dutch oven and its lid in the oven. Preheat the oven to 450°F.

- Use the additional ¼ cup bread flour and a spatula to loosen the dough from the bowl.

- Once the oven is fully heated, remove the Dutch oven, place the dough inside it, cover, and place back in the oven. Bake for 30 minutes.

- Uncover and bake for another 3 to 5 minutes, or until the bread is golden brown and fragrant. Let rest for 30 minutes and serve, or keep in a bread box for up to 3 days.

# Black Rice Pilaf

SYMPTOMS IT CAN HELP

**I** Insomnia

**W** Weight gain

SERVES 8
**Prep time:** 5 minutes
**Total time:** 50 minutes

SERVING SUGGESTION
Serve with a protein and
vegetable dish for a quick
meal.

RESET PHASE
MODIFICATIONS
**ADRENAL RESET**
**Meal:** Any
**Modification:** None

**METABOLISM RESET**
**Meal:** Dinner
**Modification:** Serve with
protein and veggies.

**THYROID RESET**
**Meal:** Any
**Modification:** None

GLUTEN-FREE OPTION
No modification needed

VEGAN OPTION
Use vegetable broth in
place of the chicken.

If you plan to use rice as a savory side dish, a pilaf can seem more
deliberate than plain rice. Black rice pairs well with beef dishes. Just use
beef broth in place of chicken or vegetable broth, or add 1 tablespoon
of tamari soy sauce.

| | | |
|---|---|---|
| Misting oil | 2 cups chicken or vegetable broth | 2 cups black rice, rinsed and drained |
| ½ cup diced onion | 1¾ cups water | |

- Coat a medium saucepan with a fine mist of oil and heat over medium-high until the oil shimmers.

- Add the onion and sauté until clear, 2 to 3 minutes. Add the broth and the water and bring to a boil. Add the rice, reduce to a simmer, and cover.

- Simmer for 30 minutes, turn off the heat, and let rest for 10 minutes. Serve immediately, or place the rice in a large covered glass storage container and refrigerate for up to 5 days.

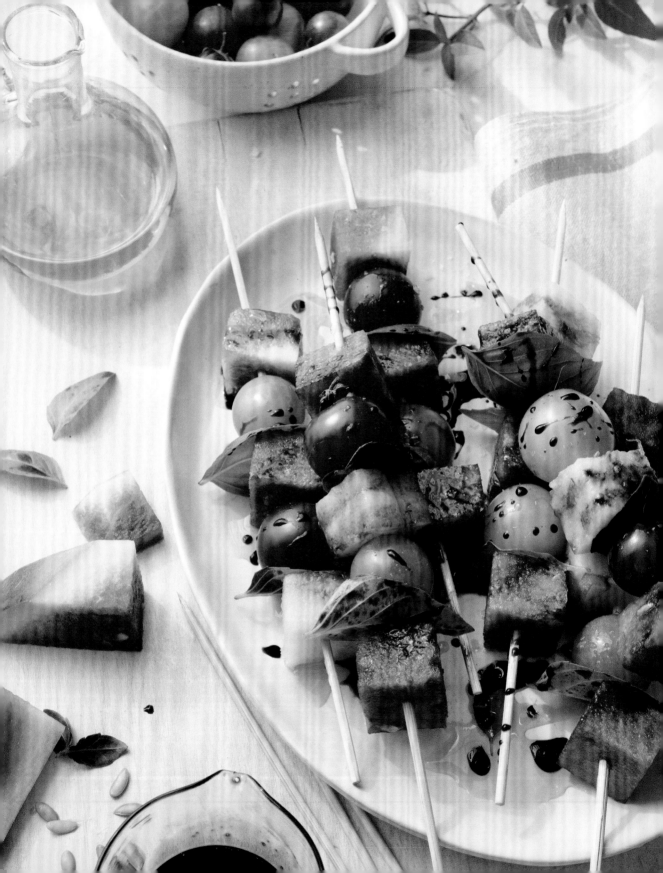

# Veggies

The evidence is incontrovertible—consuming lots of veggies leads to good health. Over the course of the day, work to have vegetables make up roughly half of your food volume. The meal plans build in variety by using different parts of the plant (roots, stems, leaves) and different families of vegetables (allium, crucifer, Apiaceae). When you plan your own menus, think about eating a variety of these categories as well as a variety of colors. Also consider a variety of cooking methods. Steamed, blanched, stir-fried, and raw are some of the best options.

**Basil, Watermelon, Tomato Skewers** 174

**Cucumber Salad with Ginger Dressing** 175

**Fig Arugula Salad** 176

**Daily Salad** 178

**Curried Almond Squash Soup** 179

**Creamy Broccoli Pistachio Soup** 181

**Gingered Collards** 182

**Seared Baby Bok Choy** 183

**Lean French Onion Soup** 185

**Kiwi Cucumber Salad** 186

**Lemony Cabbage Soup** 187

**Roasted Beet and Pistachio Salad** 188

**Roasted Root Veggies** 190

**Rosemary Cauliflower Creamed Soup** 191

**Steamed Broccoli** 192

**Beet Slaw** 193

**Sesame Coleslaw** 194

**Thai Basil Eggplant** 195

SYMPTOM KEY

 Brain fog
 Fatigue
Hot flashes
Insomnia
Weight gain

# Basil, Watermelon, Tomato Skewers

SYMPTOMS IT CAN HELP

**BF** Brain fog

**F** Fatigue

**I** Insomnia

SERVES 4
**Prep time:** 10 minutes
**Total time:** 20 minutes

RESET PHASE
MODIFICATIONS
**ADRENAL RESET**
**Meal:** Any
**Modification:** Serve in place of all other sources of carbs.

**METABOLISM RESET**
**Meal:** Dinner
**Modification:** Serve in place of all other sources of carbs.

**THYROID RESET**
**Meal:** Any
**Modification:** None

GLUTEN-FREE OPTION
No modification needed

VEGAN OPTION
No modification needed

There are several varieties of fresh basil available. Genovese and Thai are the most common, and either can work in this dish. Wait until watermelon is in season, because it needs to be both ripe and firm to hold its shape on the skewers.

¼ cup balsamic vinegar

¼ cup honey

15 bamboo skewers

1 seedless watermelon (4 to 5 pounds), cut into 30 cubes of 1 to 1½ inches

30 small basil leaves

15 ripe cherry tomatoes, halved

1 tablespoon extra-virgin olive oil

Kosher salt

■ Combine the balsamic vinegar and the honey in a small saucepan. Heat over medium heat. Bring to a simmer, stirring until the honey is dissolved, 3 to 5 minutes. Remove from heat.

■ Skewer the watermelon, basil leaves, and tomatoes, in that order. Lay the skewers on a serving platter. Drizzle the skewers with the balsamic syrup and the olive oil. Sprinkle with the salt and serve immediately as a dessert or snack.

# Cucumber Salad
# with Ginger Dressing

SYMPTOMS IT CAN HELP

HF  Hot flashes

I  Insomnia

W  Weight gain

**SERVES 4**
**Prep time:** 10 minutes
**Total time:** 10 minutes

**SERVING SUGGESTION**
Serve with a protein dish
and good carbs for a
complete meal.

**RESET PHASE
MODIFICATIONS**
**ADRENAL RESET**
**Meal:** Any
**Modification:** None

**METABOLISM RESET**
**Meal:** Any
**Modification:** None

**THYROID RESET**
**Meal:** Any
**Modification:** None

**GLUTEN-FREE OPTION**
No modification needed

**VEGAN OPTION**
No modification needed

I've always loved the house dressing served at Japanese restaurants.
It turns out that much of the flavor and texture comes from pureed
carrots! Enjoy.

**SALAD**

4 cups romaine
lettuce, washed,
dried, and torn

1 medium ripe
tomato, diced

1 cucumber, peeled,
halved lengthwise,
and sliced

2 scallions,
cleaned and sliced

**DRESSING**

¼ cup rice vinegar

¼ cup tamari
soy sauce

12 baby carrots

Juice of 1 lime

1 tablespoon honey

2 tablespoons fresh
ginger, peeled and
chopped

1 garlic clove,
minced

Kosher salt and
freshly ground
ground black
pepper to taste

- Place all the salad ingredients into a salad serving bowl and mix
  well.

- Puree the dressing ingredients in the bowl of a blender or food
  processor until smooth. Pour the dressing over the salad and serve.

# Fig Arugula Salad

HF Hot flashes

I Insomnia

W Weight gain

**SERVES 4**
**Prep time:** 15 minutes
**Total time:** 15 minutes

**SERVING SUGGESTION**
Make several hours in advance, cover, and refrigerate.

**RESET PHASE MODIFICATIONS**
**ADRENAL RESET**
**Meal:** Lunch, dinner
**Modification:** Serve with protein as a complete meal.

**METABOLISM RESET**
**Meal:** Dinner
**Modification:** Serve with protein as a complete meal.

**THYROID RESET**
**Meal:** Any
**Modification:** None

**GLUTEN-FREE OPTION**
No modification needed

**VEGAN OPTION**
No modification needed

Like beets, arugula is an excellent source of nitrate.

6 cups arugula leaves

8 figs, dried or fresh, stems removed and cut into quarters

1 teaspoon folic-acid-free nutritional yeast

2 tablespoons pine nuts

2 tablespoons honey

2 tablespoons balsamic vinegar

1 tablespoon extra-virgin olive oil

- Combine all the ingredients in a large serving bowl and stir.

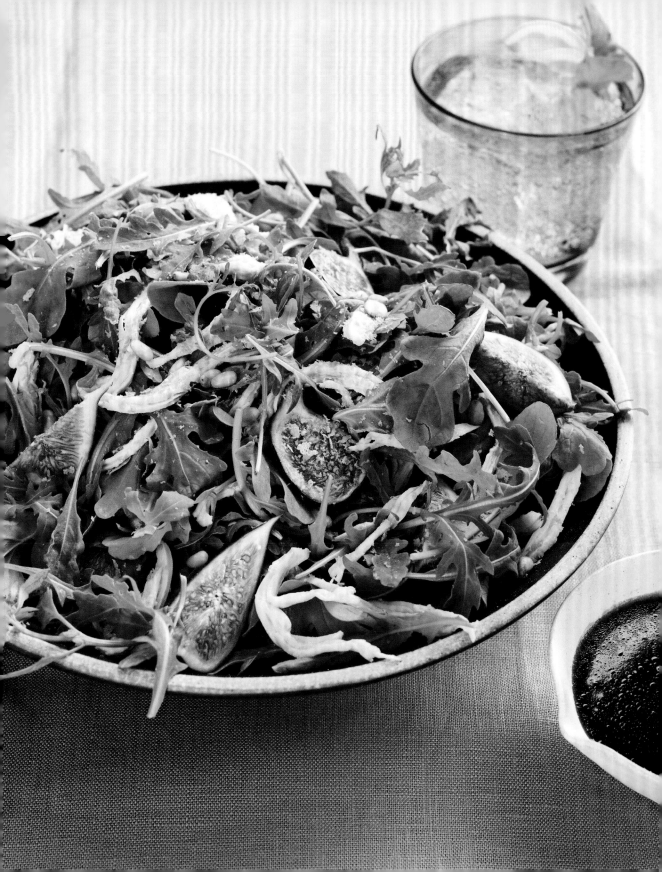

# Daily Salad

(BF) Brain fog

(F) Fatigue

(HF) Hot flashes

(I) Insomnia

(W) Weight gain

SERVES 4
**Prep time:** 10 minutes
**Total time:** 10 minutes

I've laid out an easy template for a daily salad. Feel free to mix veggies based on what you have on hand.

4 cups salad greens: washed and torn leaves of spinach, romaine lettuce, red leaf lettuce, green leaf lettuce, butter lettuce, or other leafy greens

Additions: cherry tomatoes, diced cucumber, shaved onion, shredded carrot, shredded beets, diced jicama, sliced radish

- Wash and dry all ingredients. Cut or tear to desired serving sizes. Combine in a salad bowl, add any dressing (see below), and serve as a vegetable dish.

- FOR DRESSING: Combine 1 to 2 teaspoons olive oil or neutral oil, 1 to 2 tablespoons balsamic or apple cider vinegar, and salt and pepper to taste.

  OR

- SAVORY DRESSING RECIPE: Combine 1 tablespoon maple syrup, 1 tablespoon olive oil, 2 tablespoons apple cider vinegar, 1 tablespoon Dijon mustard, and 1 clove of minced garlic.

- ASIAN DRESSING RECIPE: Combine 1 tablespoon tamari soy sauce, 1 teaspoon toasted sesame oil, and 2 tablespoons seasoned rice vinegar.

# Curried Almond Squash Soup

**SERVES 4**
**Prep time:** 10 minutes
**Total time:** 70 minutes

**SERVING SUGGESTION**
Serve with a protein dish
for a complete meal.

**RESET PHASE
MODIFICATIONS**
**ADRENAL RESET**
**Meal:** Any
**Modification:** Serve with
a source of protein.

**METABOLISM RESET**
**Meal:** Dinner
**Modification:** Serve with
a source of protein.

**THYROID RESET**
**Meal:** Any
**Modification:** None

**GLUTEN-FREE OPTION**
No modification needed

**VEGAN OPTIONS**
No modification needed

Kabocha, also called Japanese pumpkin, is a hard winter squash. The flavor is sweeter and more pronounced than that of other squashes. If you can't find kabocha squash, butternut or acorn squash can be used. For the nondairy milk, flax milk or coconut milk will work well in this recipe. You may find that your blender heats the mixture so much that it will be hot enough to serve. If not, add it to a saucepan and warm to serve.

1 kabocha squash (2 to 3 pounds), seeded and sliced into quarters

One 2-inch section fresh ginger, peeled and sliced

1 sweet or yellow onion, diced

¼ cup whole almonds or almond flour

4 cups vegetable broth

¾ cup nondairy milk of choice

1 tablespoon curry powder

- Preheat the oven to 350°F.

- Place the sliced squash on a baking pan with the cut side up. Drape the ginger slices and the onion over the squash and bake for 50 minutes, until the squash is fork-tender. Remove from the oven and allow to cool for 10 minutes. Once the squash has cooled, scoop the flesh out of the skin and discard the skin.

- If using whole almonds, place them in the bowl of a high-speed blender and blend on high until flour is formed. Add the vegetables, almond flour, vegetable broth, nondairy milk, and curry powder and blend, loosely covered, for 2 minutes. Work in batches if needed.

- Heat and serve immediately, or refrigerate for a later meal.

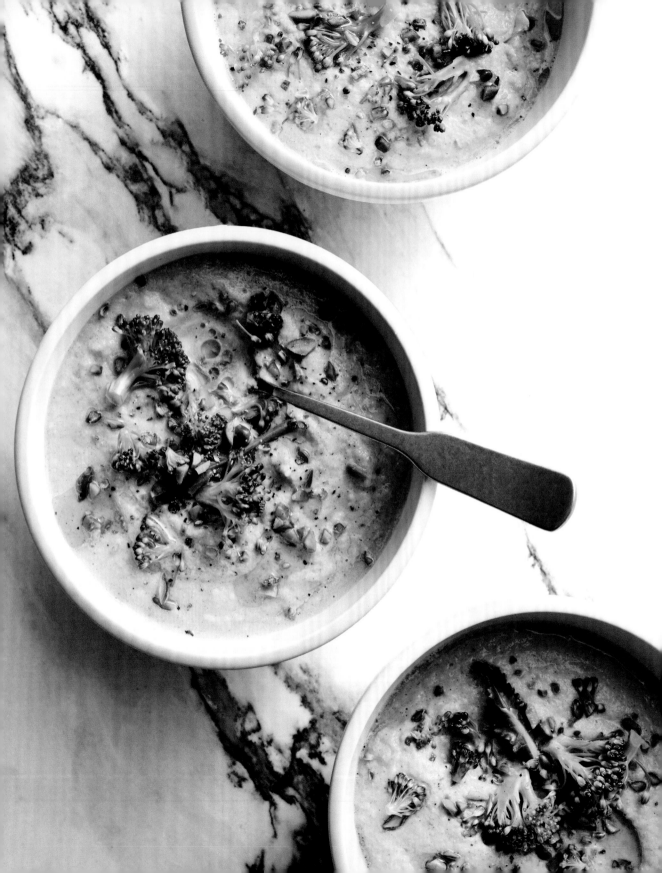

# Creamy Broccoli Pistachio Soup

## SYMPTOMS IT CAN HELP

**BF** Brain fog

**HF** Hot flashes

**I** Insomnia

## SERVES 4
**Prep time:** 5 minutes
**Total time:** 15 minutes

## SERVING SUGGESTION
Serve with good carbs and protein for a complete meal.

## RESET PHASE MODIFICATIONS
**ADRENAL RESET**
**Meal:** Any
**Modification:** Serve in place of other fats.

**METABOLISM RESET**
**Meal:** Dinner
**Modification:** Serve in place of other fats.

**THYROID RESET**
**Meal:** Any
**Modification:** None

## GLUTEN-FREE OPTION
No modification needed

## VEGAN OPTION
Use vegetable stock instead of chicken stock.

Creamy soups are usually full of empty calories and fat. Not this one! Pistachios and broccoli pair to create an excellent flavor and rich texture. Be careful with a blender and hot ingredients. Only fill the blender a fourth or a third full, and do not cover too tightly. You can use salted or unsalted pistachios, but consider using less salt to taste when using salted pistachios.

Misting oil

⅓ cup shelled pistachios

1 medium onion, diced

4 cups broccoli florets and chopped stems

2 cups chicken stock

1 cup water

Kosher salt and freshly ground black pepper to taste

- Mist a medium saucepan with the oil and heat on medium-high until the oil shimmers. If the pistachios are raw, sauté them for 1 to 2 minutes, until fragrant. You can skip this step if they are toasted.

- Add the onion and sauté for 2 to 3 minutes until it softens. Add the broccoli and sauté an additional 3 to 5 minutes until it softens as well. Remove a few large spoonfuls of broccoli and pistachios for garnish.

- Add in the stock and the water. Bring to a simmer and cook for 5 minutes, stirring occasionally. Add salt and pepper to taste. Puree using a blender or immersion blender.

- To serve, pour the soup into bowls and sprinkle with the reserved broccoli and pistachios.

# Gingered Collards

## SYMPTOMS IT CAN HELP

BF Brain fog

I Insomnia

W Weight gain

**SERVES 4**
**Prep time:** 3 minutes
**Total time:** 20 minutes

**SERVING SUGGESTION**
Serve as the main or secondary vegetable dish with any meal.

**RESET PHASE MODIFICATIONS**
**ADRENAL RESET**
**Meal:** Any
**Modification:** None

**METABOLISM RESET**
**Meal:** Any
**Modification:** None

**THYROID RESET**
**Meal:** Any
**Modification:** None

**GLUTEN-FREE OPTION**
No modification needed

**VEGAN OPTION**
No modification needed

Kale has had too much attention these last few years, and poor collard greens have been ignored. Not in this cookbook!

1 tablespoon olive oil

2 tablespoons freshly grated ginger

2 cloves garlic, minced

1 bunch of collard greens, rinsed, stemmed, and cut into 1-inch strips

½ cup vegetable stock

1 tablespoon sesame seeds, dry toasted until light brown

Finishing salt, such as Maldon Sea Salt

- Add the olive oil to a medium sauté pan and heat on medium for 30 seconds. Add the ginger and the garlic and stir for an additional 30 seconds, or until the garlic becomes soft.

- Add the collard greens and the vegetable stock to the pan and raise the heat to high. Cover and cook 5 to 7 minutes, until the collards are soft but still green.

- Uncover and continue to cook until the liquid has evaporated, roughly 1 to 2 more minutes.

- Stir in the sesame seeds. Sprinkle on the finishing salt immediately before serving.

# Seared Baby Bok Choy

HF  Hot flashes

I  Insomnia

W  Weight gain

**SERVES 4**
**Prep time:** 4 minutes
**Total time:** 10 minutes

**SERVING SUGGESTION**
Serve with protein and a healthy carb.

**RESET PHASE MODIFICATIONS**
**ADRENAL RESET**
**Meal:** Any
**Modification:** None

**METABOLISM RESET**
**Meal:** Any
**Modification:** None

**THYROID RESET**
**Meal:** Any
**Modification:** None

**GLUTEN-FREE OPTION**
No modification needed

**VEGAN OPTION**
No modification needed

Here is my all-time favorite vegetable! I like bok choy as well, but baby bok choy has an even milder taste and thinner stalks that cook up into a less watery texture. Stainless steel or cast-iron pans work best for searing. Be sure to get your oiled pan nice and hot before adding the bok choy.

3 tablespoons white miso paste

1 teaspoon extra-virgin olive oil

1 tablespoon fresh lemon juice

Misting oil

1½ pounds baby bok choy (4 to 5 bunches), ends trimmed and cut in half lengthwise

Kosher salt and freshly ground black pepper to taste

- To make the dressing, stir the miso, oil, and lemon juice together in a small bowl.

- Heat a 12-inch skillet on high and mist with the oil. Lay the bok choy in the skillet, cut side down, and drizzle with about half the dressing. Work in batches if needed.

- Sear the bok choy for 2 to 3 minutes, then turn and sear for another minute, adding the remainder of the dressing plus the salt and pepper.

- Remove from heat and serve immediately.

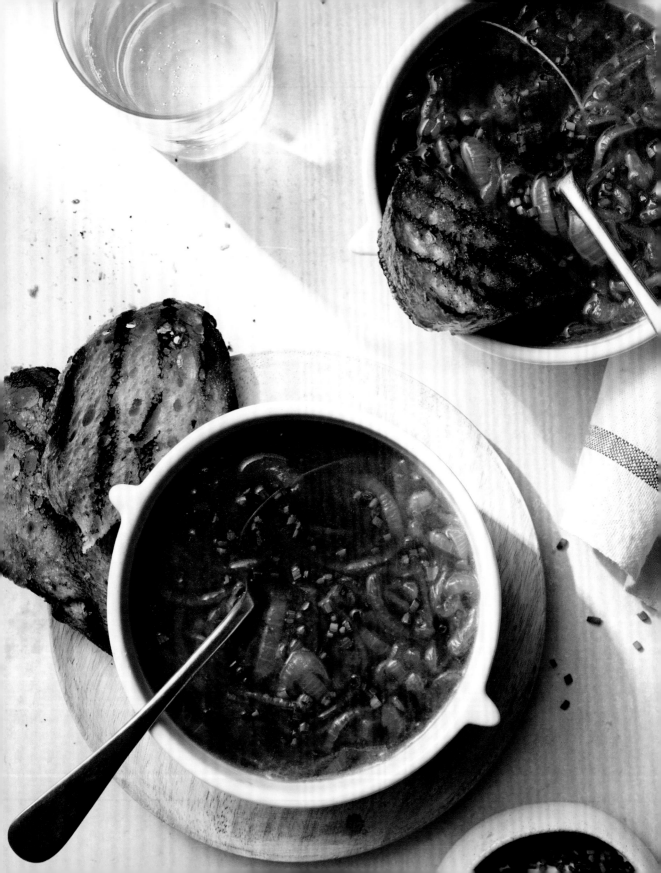

# Lean French Onion Soup

SYMPTOMS IT CAN HELP

**F** Fatigue

**I** Insomnia

**W** Weight gain

**SERVES 4**
**Prep time:** 5 minutes
**Total time:** 1 hour

**RESET PHASE
MODIFICATIONS**
**ADRENAL RESET**
**Meal:** Any
**Modification:** Serve with
protein and good carbs.

**METABOLISM RESET**
**Meal:** Dinner
**Modification:** Serve in
place of other carbs.

**THYROID RESET**
**Meal:** Any
**Modification:** None

**GLUTEN-FREE OPTION**
Use a gluten-free
all-purpose flour like
Bob's Red Mill.

**VEGAN OPTION**
Substitute vegetable
broth for beef broth.

I can't imagine a better way to get a whopping dose of onions all at once. However, most French onion soup recipes use more than a stick of butter per pot of soup. Here is a simplified and lightened-up version that many have come to prefer over restaurant-style French onion. I like to serve it as is, rather than adding bread and cheese on top. This recipe calls for yellow onions, but you can also use sweet Vidalia onions. Use a homemade beef broth, or one you know you like. My favorite is the Better Than Bouillon brand.

1 teaspoon
neutral oil

2½ pounds yellow
onions, thinly sliced

2 tablespoons
all-purpose flour

3 ounces
dry white wine

1 bay leaf

10 cups beef broth

Kosher salt and
freshly ground black
pepper to taste

- Heat the oil in a large stockpot on medium until it starts to shimmer.

- Reduce the heat to medium-low and add the onions. Stir frequently and sauté for 20 to 30 minutes, or until lightly caramelized. Add ½ teaspoon of the beef broth if they start to stick.

- Add the flour to the onions. Mix well and sauté for another 3 minutes. Add the wine and the bay leaf. Bring the mixture to a simmer and cook for 10 minutes.

- Add the beef broth and the salt and pepper. Cover the pot and simmer for 20 minutes.

- Ladle into serving bowls and let cool, uncovered, for 5 minutes prior to serving.

# Kiwi Cucumber Salad

**SERVES 4**
**Prep time:** 10 minutes
**Total time:**10 minutes

**SERVING SUGGESTION**
Serve with a light protein dish and sourdough, or with a side of warmed cannellini beans.

**RESET PHASE MODIFICATIONS**
**ADRENAL RESET**
**Meal:** Any
**Modification:** None

**METABOLISM RESET**
**Meal:** Dinner
**Modification:** Serve with a carb and protein without additional fat.

**THYROID RESET**
**Meal:** Any
**Modification:** None

**GLUTEN-FREE OPTION**
No modification needed

**VEGAN OPTION**
No modification needed

This salad is delicious! The lime zest is important. This recipe does best with kiwi that is soft to the touch but not overripe. Use the freshest mint sprigs and save the rest for tea or other dishes.

1 head romaine lettuce, washed and torn

6 kiwifruit, peeled and diced

½ long English cucumber, sliced thin

⅓ cup crushed walnut pieces

10 mint sprigs

¼ cup extra-virgin olive oil

1 tablespoon fresh lime juice

1 teaspoon lime zest

¼ cup rice vinegar or white vinegar

2 teaspoons honey

Kosher salt and freshly ground black pepper to taste

Optional: ⅓ cup pomegranate arils

- Place the lettuce in a salad serving bowl. Top with the kiwi, cucumber, and walnut pieces. Remove the mint leaves from sprigs and add to the salad.

- In a small bowl, whisk the olive oil, lime juice, lime zest, vinegar, honey, and salt and pepper into a vinaigrette.

- Pour the vinaigrette over the salad. Top with the pomegranate arils, if using. Season to taste and serve immediately.

# Lemony Cabbage Soup

SYMPTOMS IT CAN HELP

**HF** Hot flashes

**I** Insomnia

**W** Weight gain

SERVES 4
**Prep time:** 15 minutes
**Total time:** 30 minutes

SERVING SUGGESTION
Serve with carbs and protein for a complete meal.

RESET PHASE MODIFICATIONS
**ADRENAL RESET**
**Meal:** Lunch, dinner
**Modification:** None

**METABOLISM RESET**
**Meal:** Any
**Modification:** None

**THYROID RESET**
**Meal:** Any
**Modification:** None

GLUTEN-FREE OPTION
No modification needed

VEGAN OPTION
No modification needed

Cabbage is a rich source of sulfur compounds that help skin and hair. It also has glutamine derivatives that soothe digestion. If you are old enough, you might remember when cabbage soup was a magic food for weight loss. There is enough good evidence for its benefits that it no longer needs to hide behind magic!

Misting oil

1 onion, diced

1 cup baby carrots, halved

2 celery stalks, diced

2 cloves garlic, minced

1 teaspoon dried oregano

½ medium head cabbage, shredded

2 teaspoons kosher salt

1 (14-ounce) can diced tomatoes

4 cups vegetable broth

2 tablespoons fresh lemon juice

2 teaspoons lemon zest

¼ cup chopped fresh parsley

Freshly ground black pepper to taste

- Mist a stockpot with a fine spray of oil and heat on medium-high until the oil starts to shimmer.

- Sauté the onion for 1 minute, until it starts to soften. Add the carrots, celery, garlic, and oregano. Sauté an additional 2 to 4 minutes, until the carrots soften. Add the cabbage and sauté 2 minutes, or until it softens as well.

- Add the salt, tomatoes (including liquid), and vegetable broth. Bring to a simmer and let cook, uncovered, for 10 minutes. Remove from heat and add the lemon juice, lemon zest, parsley, and pepper. Serve immediately.

# Roasted Beet and Pistachio Salad

## SYMPTOMS IT CAN HELP

F Fatigue

I Insomnia

W Weight gain

## SERVES 4
**Prep time:** 40 minutes
**Total time:** 60 minutes

## SERVING SUGGESTION
Make this several hours in advance, cover, and refrigerate.

## RESET PHASE MODIFICATIONS
**ADRENAL RESET**
**Meal:** Any
**Modification:** None

**METABOLISM RESET**
**Meal:** Dinner
**Modification:** Serve with protein and no additional fats.

**THYROID RESET**
**Meal:** Any
**Modification:** None

## GLUTEN-FREE OPTION
No modification needed

## VEGAN OPTION
No modification needed

This is an excellent salad for entertaining or to serve as the centerpiece of a meal. I mostly make it when we have leftover roasted beets or precooked beets from the supermarket.

8 medium or 4 large beets, peeled and cut into 1-inch wedges

3 garlic cloves, minced

Misting oil

⅓ cup unsalted toasted pistachios

2 cups baby spinach leaves

¼ cup rice vinegar

1 tablespoon extra-virgin olive oil

Kosher salt and freshly ground black pepper to taste

- Preheat the oven to 350°F.

- In a medium bowl, toss the beets with the garlic and a mist of oil. Pour into a baking dish and lightly cover with foil. Bake for 30 minutes, or until the beets are tender. Let sit for 15 minutes until cool.

- In a salad bowl, combine the cooked beets with the pistachios, spinach leaves, vinegar, olive oil, and salt and pepper to taste.

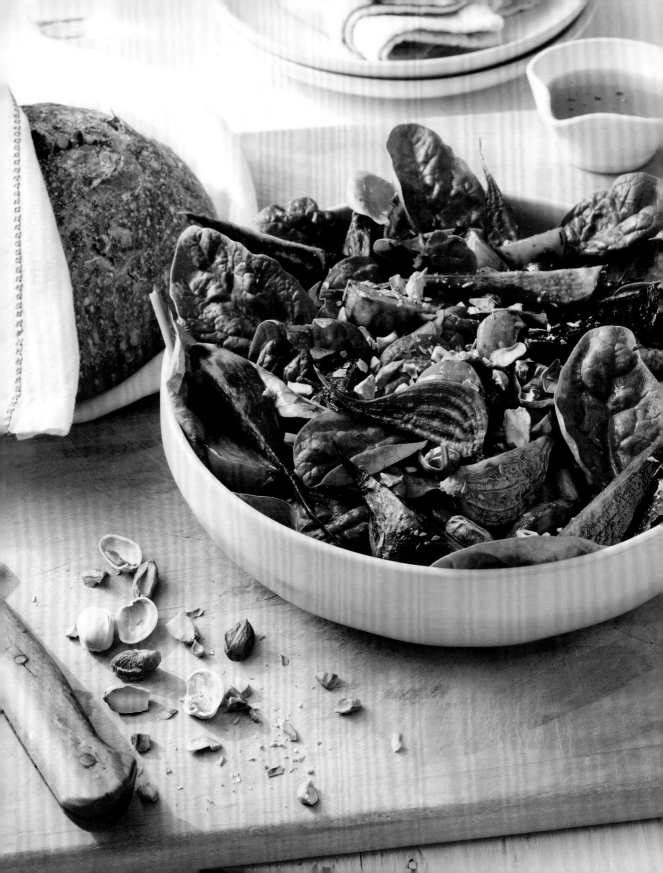

# Roasted Root Veggies

This is a nice side dish to have prepped in advance. You can precook it and heat it when ready, but my first choice is to have it prepped and ready to go in the oven and roast it when needed. The best options for the vegetables include beets, carrots, celery root, fennel, parsnips, potatoes, rutabagas, sweet potatoes, and turnips.

**SYMPTOMS IT CAN HELP**

BF Brain fog

F Fatigue

HF Hot flashes

I Insomnia

W Weight gain

**SERVES 8**
**Prep time:** 10 minutes
**Total time:** 40 minutes

**SERVING SUGGESTIONS**
Serve with protein and good carbs for a complete meal.

**RESET PHASE MODIFICATIONS**
**ADRENAL RESET**
**Meal:** Any
**Modification:** None

**METABOLISM RESET**
**Meal:** Dinner
**Modification:** Serve with protein and no additional fats.

**THYROID RESET**
**Meal:** Any
**Modification:** None

**GLUTEN-FREE OPTION**
No modification needed

**VEGAN OPTION**
No modification needed

6 cups peeled and roughly chopped (1- to 2-inch pieces) root vegetables

Kosher salt to taste

- Preheat the oven to 400°F and cover a baking pan with parchment paper.

- Add the veggies to the pan, spread them out evenly, and sprinkle with the salt. Place in the oven and bake for 35 to 40 minutes, until lightly browned (or let them go a bit longer if you like them crispier), checking and stirring every 10 minutes.

- Serve or refrigerate for up to 3 days.

# Rosemary Cauliflower Creamed Soup

The flavors of rosemary can be intense if not buffered by other ingredients. Rosemary oil is one solution to this issue. Use lightly flavored olive oil or even a neutral oil to make it.

Misting oil

1 medium onion, chopped

2 garlic cloves, minced

4 cups chicken stock

4 (3- to 5-inch) sprigs fresh rosemary

1 head cauliflower, cored

2 teaspoons kosher salt

Freshly ground black pepper to taste

- Mist a stockpot with a fine spray of oil and heat on medium-high until the oil starts to shimmer. Sauté the onion for 1 minute, until it starts to soften. Add the garlic and sauté an additional 2 minutes.

- Add the chicken stock, rosemary sprigs, cauliflower, salt, and pepper and bring to a gentle boil. Reduce heat and lightly simmer for 12 to 15 minutes, until the cauliflower is tender.

- Remove the rosemary sprigs and, using a blender or an immersion blender, puree the soup, leaving roughly a fourth of it unpureed for texture. Serve immediately.

# Steamed Broccoli

## SYMPTOMS IT CAN HELP

**BF** Brain fog

**F** Fatigue

**HF** Hot flashes

**I** Insomnia

**W** Weight gain

**SERVES 8**
**Prep time:** 5 minutes
**Total time:** 15 minutes

## RESET PHASE MODIFICATIONS

**ADRENAL RESET**
**Meal:** Any
**Modification:** Serve with good carbs and protein.

**METABOLISM RESET**
**Meal:** Dinner
**Modification:** Serve with good carbs and protein.

**THYROID RESET**
**Meal:** Any
**Modification:** None

I used broccoli in this recipe, but feel free to use a wide range of vegetables. Some good options include frozen mixed veggies, parsnips, broccoli rabe, cauliflower, carrots, zucchini, Brussels sprouts, or some combination. You can also combine several types. Just add them in at different stages if their cooking times differ. When batch-cooking vegetables, you want to leave them a bit undercooked. That way when you reheat them to serve, they will not be overdone.

1 quart water

2 tablespoons kosher salt

2 large bunches of broccoli (2 pounds), florets and peeled stems, cut into pieces ½ to 1 inch in size

- In a 6-quart stockpot with a steamer basket, bring the water to a boil and add the salt. Place the broccoli in the steamer basket, lower it into the pot, and cover.

- Steam for 3 to 4 minutes. Lift the steamer basket out and rinse the broccoli under cold water for 30 seconds to stop the cooking.

- Let cool for 10 minutes. Serve or refrigerate for up to 5 days.

# Beet Slaw

BF Brain fog

F Fatigue

W Weight gain

**SERVES 4**
**Prep time:** 5 minutes
**Total time:** 5 minutes

**SERVING SUGGESTION**
Make several hours in
advance, cover, and
refrigerate.

**RESET PHASE
MODIFICATIONS**
**ADRENAL RESET**
**Meal:** Any
**Modification:** None

**METABOLISM RESET**
**Meal:** Any–unlimited
food
**Modification:** None

**THYROID RESET**
**Meal:** Any
**Modification:** None

**GLUTEN-FREE OPTION**
No modification needed

**VEGAN OPTION**
No modification needed

Promise me that you won't overthink this one. Something this good *can* be this easy. It's worth having some rubber gloves on hand for dishes like this unless you don't mind getting caught red-handed (excuse the pun).

Juice of 1 lemon

2 teaspoons Sucanat or natural sweetener of choice

½ teaspoon kosher salt

1 teaspoon extra-virgin olive oil

2 medium beets, peeled and shredded with a box shredder or food processor

- Whisk the lemon juice, Sucanat, salt, and oil in a small bowl. Place the shredded beets in a salad bowl and mix in the dressing.

- Serve and enjoy!

# Sesame Coleslaw

SYMPTOMS IT CAN HELP

BF Brain fog

HF Hot flashes

I Insomnia

SERVES 4
**Prep time:** 10 minutes
**Total time:** 10 minutes

SERVING SUGGESTION
Make several hours in
advance, cover, and
refrigerate.

RESET PHASE
MODIFICATIONS
**ADRENAL RESET**
**Meal:** Lunch, dinner
**Modification:** None

**METABOLISM RESET**
**Meal:** Any
**Modification:** None

**THYROID RESET**
**Meal:** Any
**Modification:** None

GLUTEN-FREE OPTION
No modification needed

VEGAN OPTION
No modification needed

This is the perfect way to easily get in your greens and cruciferous veggies. It is especially fast if you're using a food processor or purchasing a coleslaw mix that has already been prepped.

**SALAD**

¼ head cabbage, shredded

1 large carrot, grated

½ red onion, thinly sliced

**DRESSING**

1 teaspoon toasted sesame oil

1 tablespoon sesame seeds

1 tablespoon tamari soy sauce

Juice of 2 limes

- Combine the salad ingredients in a large serving bowl.

- Whisk the dressing ingredients together in a small bowl. Pour over the salad and stir thoroughly.

- Serve and enjoy!

# Thai Basil Eggplant

## SYMPTOMS IT CAN HELP

BF Brain fog

F Fatigue

W Weight gain

**SERVES 4**
**Prep time:** 10 minutes
**Total time:** 20 minutes

**SERVING SUGGESTION**
Serve over rice and along with protein such as cooked chicken or tofu.

**RESET PHASE MODIFICATIONS**
**ADRENAL RESET**
**Meal:** Any
**Modification:** None

**METABOLISM RESET**
**Meal:** Dinner
**Modification:** Serve in place of all other sources of fat.

**THYROID RESET**
**Meal:** Any
**Modification:** None

**GLUTEN-FREE OPTION**
No modification needed

**VEGAN OPTION**
No modification needed

Thai basil is a more aromatic form of basil with similar health benefits. Try it if you can find it, but don't worry if you only have regular basil. You can use Italian eggplants in place of the Japanese eggplants, but if you do, be sure to peel them first.

Misting oil

2 Japanese eggplants cut on an angle into 1½-inch wedges

3 cloves garlic, minced

3 scallions, sliced

4 ounces Thai basil or holy basil leaves (about 1 cup loosely packed)

1 teaspoon cornstarch or arrowroot powder

1 tablespoon white cooking wine

2 teaspoons fish sauce

½ teaspoon Sucanat or natural sweetener of choice

2 teaspoons tamari soy sauce

1 teaspoon toasted sesame oil

½ teaspoon ground white pepper

¼ cup vegetable stock

- Mist a wok or large skillet with the oil and heat on medium-high. Spread the eggplant out evenly and sear, covered, for 2 minutes. Uncover, turn the eggplant, and sear for another 2 minutes.

- Turn again, raise the heat to high, and cook a final 1 to 2 minutes, until the eggplant is a golden-brown color. Transfer to a bowl.

- Mist the wok again with oil and add the garlic, scallions, and basil. Stir-fry for 30 seconds and add the eggplant back in.

- Add all the remaining ingredients and stir until well combined, smooth, and heated, roughly 1 to 2 minutes. Serve immediately.

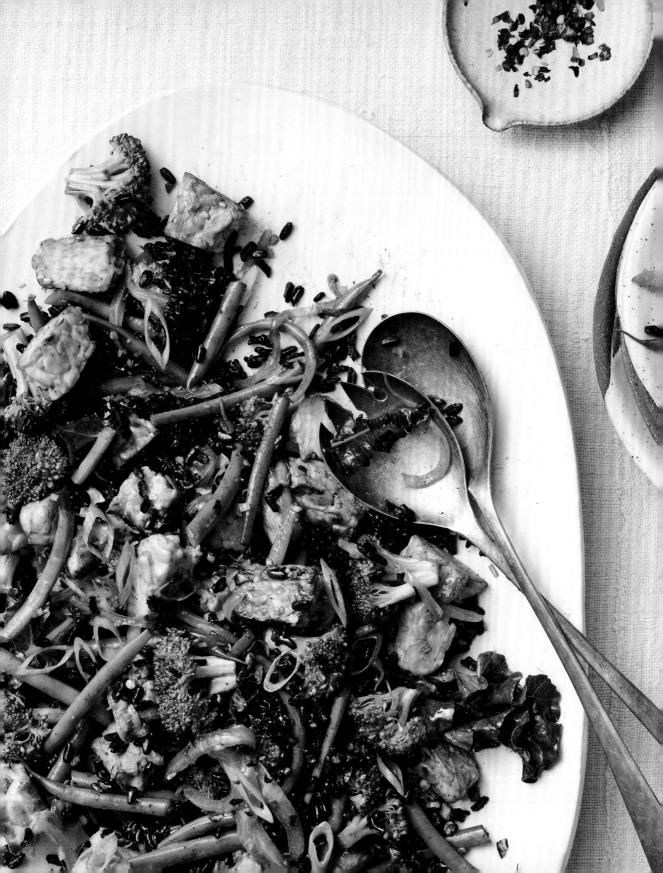

# Main Dishes

Main dishes are complete meals including veggies, protein, and healthy carbs. You'll find a nice mix of options here—from hearty proteins with delicious sides to soups, stir-fries, salads, and more—to serve as a satisfying and delicious lunch or dinner.

**Forbidden Tempeh Rice** 198

**Curried Eggplant, Chickpeas, and Tomatoes** 201

**Cactus Chili** 202

**Ginger Garlic Stir-Fry** 204

**Green Chili with Chicken** 205

**Foil-Baked Chicken and Radishes** 206

**Healthy Niçoise Salad** 209

**Lentil Veggie Soup** 210

**Minestrone Meatloaf** 211

**Shrimp and Spicy Rice Noodles** 213

**Tofu Veggie Laksa** 214

SYMPTOM KEY

- BF Brain fog
- F Fatigue
- HF Hot flashes
- I Insomnia
- W Weight gain

# Forbidden Tempeh Rice

SYMPTOMS IT CAN HELP

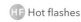 Hot flashes

I Insomnia

**SERVES 4**
**Prep time:** 10 minutes
**Total time:** 20 minutes

RESET PHASE
MODIFICATIONS
**ADRENAL RESET**
**Meal:** Any
**Modification:** None

**METABOLISM RESET**
**Meal:** Dinner
**Modification:** None

**THYROID RESET**
**Meal:** Any
**Modification:** None

GLUTEN-FREE OPTION
No modification needed

VEGAN OPTION
No modification needed

Black rice is the star of this stir-fry. Tempeh is a traditional fermented food first used in Indonesian cuisines. It is a complete protein and rich in fiber, micronutrients, prebiotics, and antioxidants. Most large supermarkets carry it in the refrigerated or frozen food section. Be sure the rice is refrigerated, and don't stir too much after you add it in. Otherwise, the colors of the other ingredients will be lost.

Misting oil

1 (12-ounce) package tempeh, thawed and cut into bite-size pieces

2 stalks fresh lemongrass, with root and outer leaves discarded and white section finely chopped, or 2 tablespoons dried lemongrass

2 cloves garlic, minced

¼ cup water

1 head broccoli, cut into bite-size pieces, stems removed

1 pound green beans, cut into 2-inch sections

1 medium onion, sliced

1 tablespoon honey

½ to 1 teaspoon red chili flakes (adjust per heat tolerance)

2 tablespoons tamari soy sauce

2 cups cooked black rice, refrigerated

2 scallions, coarsely chopped

- Mist the oil in a wok or large skillet and heat on medium until a drop of water sizzles.

- Add the tempeh and sauté until it starts to brown, roughly 5 minutes. Add the lemongrass and garlic and sauté an additional 2 minutes.

- Add the water, broccoli, green beans, onion, honey, chili flakes, and tamari. Sauté an additional 5 minutes, or until the vegetables are cooked and colorful.

- Add the black rice and stir until it is just heated. Garnish with the scallions and serve.

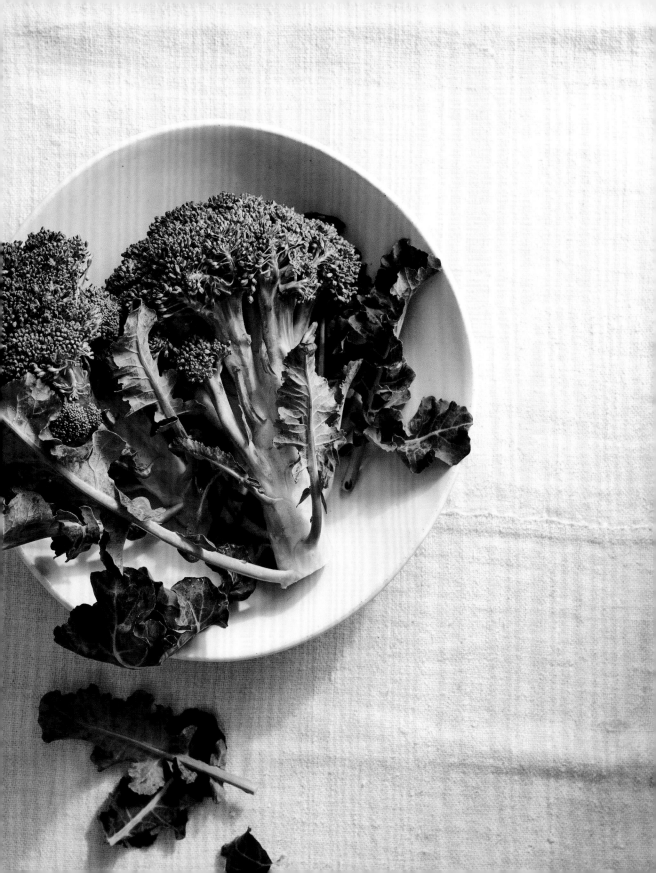

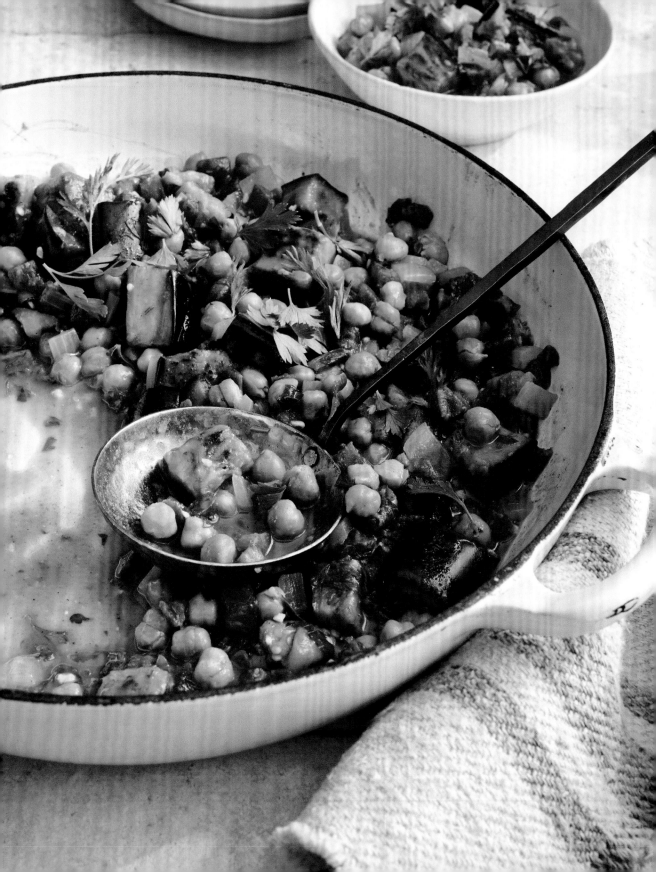

# Curried Eggplant, Chickpeas, and Tomatoes

SYMPTOMS IT CAN HELP

BF Brain fog

HF Hot flashes

I Insomnia

SERVES 4
**Prep time:** 30 minutes
**Total time:** 45 minutes

SERVING SUGGESTION
Serve as a complete meal.

RESET PHASE
MODIFICATIONS
**ADRENAL RESET**
**Meal:** Any
**Modification:** None

**METABOLISM RESET**
**Meal:** Dinner
**Modification:** Serve
with a carb and without
additional fat.

**THYROID RESET**
**Meal:** Any
**Modification:** None

GLUTEN-FREE OPTION
No modification needed

VEGAN OPTION
No modification needed

For this dish, feel free to use an Asian eggplant if that's what you have on hand.

Misting oil

1 eggplant, rinsed, stem removed, and cubed

Kosher salt to taste

1 medium onion, diced

1 tablespoon peeled and minced fresh ginger

3 cloves garlic, minced

1 tablespoon curry powder

1 (13.5-ounce) can light coconut milk

1 (14.5-ounce) can diced tomatoes, drained

1 (14.5-ounce) can chickpeas, drained

Garnish: ½ cup chopped fresh parsley leaves

- Preheat the oven to 400°F.

- Lightly mist a baking pan with the oil. Lay out the diced eggplant on it, apply another mist of oil to it, and sprinkle with the salt. Bake for 25 minutes, stirring every 5 minutes.

- While the eggplant is cooking, mist a medium saucepan with the oil and heat on medium until the oil shimmers. Add the onion, ginger, and garlic. Sauté for 3 to 4 minutes, stirring frequently.

- Add the curry powder and sauté for an additional 2 minutes, stirring frequently. Add in the coconut milk, tomatoes, roasted eggplant, and chickpeas. Bring to a low simmer and cook until the eggplant is soft, roughly 3 to 5 minutes. Garnish with the parsley and serve.

# Cactus Chili

SYMPTOMS IT CAN HELP

F Fatigue

I Insomnia

W Weight gain

SERVES 4
**Prep time:** 15 minutes
**Total time:** 45 minutes

RESET PHASE
MODIFICATIONS
**ADRENAL RESET**
**Meal:** Any
**Modification:** None

**METABOLISM RESET**
**Meal:** Dinner
**Modification:** None

**THYROID RESET**
**Meal:** Any
**Modification:** None

GLUTEN-FREE OPTION
No modification needed

VEGAN OPTION
Substitute crumbled
tempeh for beef.

Yup, it's really cactus. Prickly pear leaves are one of the richest known sources of soluble fiber. They do an amazing job of stabilizing blood sugar and reducing appetite. With the addition of cayenne, this dish is a great weight-loss recipe. As exotic as cactus sounds, it is easy to find. Most supermarkets have canned nopalitos in the Mexican food section. If you can't find them, consider fresh or frozen okra as a good substitute.

1 pound lean (97%) ground beef

1 medium yellow onion, diced

4 cloves garlic, minced

1 (15-ounce) jar nopalitos

1 tablespoon ground cumin

4 tablespoons chili powder

1 teaspoon cayenne pepper (less if you're sensitive to heat)

1 (14.5-ounce) can diced tomatoes with liquid

2 tablespoons tomato paste

1 (14.5-ounce) can kidney beans with liquid

1½ teaspoons kosher salt

¼ teaspoon freshly ground black pepper

4 cups spinach leaves

- Brown the beef in a 4- to 6-quart saucepan over medium heat for roughly 5 minutes and drain thoroughly.

- Add the onion and garlic and sauté with the beef for 2 to 3 minutes, or until the onion softens. Add the nopalitos, cumin, chili powder, cayenne, diced tomatoes, tomato paste, kidney beans, salt, and black pepper.

- Simmer, lightly covered, on low for 40 minutes. Add in the spinach leaves and stir until wilted and incorporated. Serve as a complete meal.

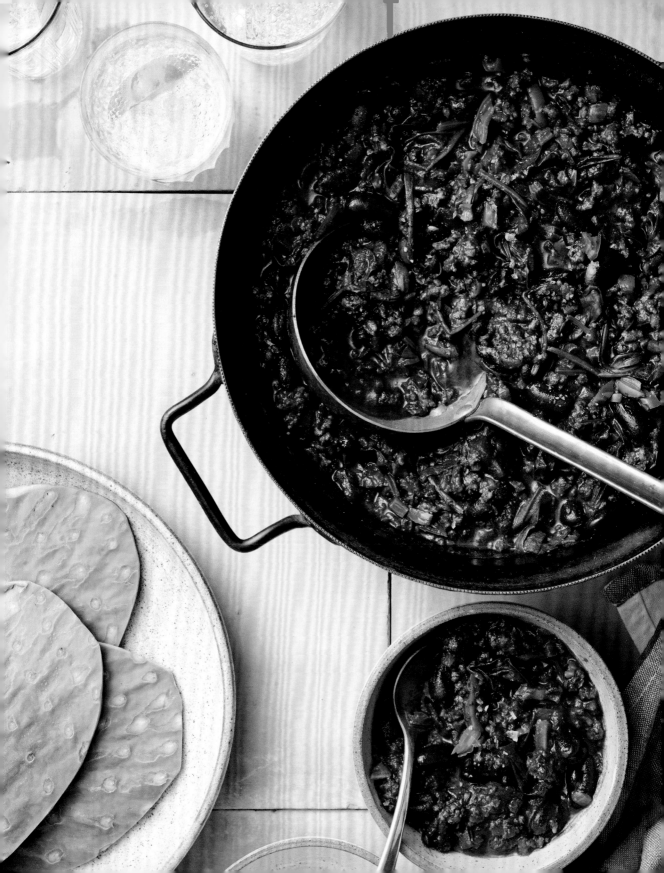

# Ginger Garlic Stir-Fry

This is the quintessential veggie stir-fry. Feel free to mix and match with other veggies. This dish is great to make when you have an odd hodgepodge of veggies left in the fridge, because nearly any combination can work. This recipe is also a good lesson in how to stir-fry without bathing the food in oil.

## SYMPTOMS IT CAN HELP

BF Brain fog

F Fatigue

W Weight gain

## SERVES 4
**Prep time:** 10 minutes
**Total time:** 20 minutes

## SERVING SUGGESTION
Serve over rice.

## RESET PHASE MODIFICATIONS
**ADRENAL RESET**
**Meal:** Any
**Modification:** None

**METABOLISM RESET**
**Meal:** Dinner
**Modification:** None

**THYROID RESET**
**Meal:** Any
**Modification:** None

## GLUTEN-FREE OPTION
No modification needed

## VEGAN OPTION
Omit the chicken and use 2 (12-ounce) packages of tempeh, cut into bite-size pieces.

Misting oil

1 tablespoon cornstarch or arrowroot powder

2 tablespoons gluten-free soy sauce

2 tablespoons vegetable broth or water

1 cup sliced white button mushrooms

¼ cup diced onion

1 small head broccoli, cut into florets

2 teaspoons peeled and minced fresh ginger, divided

3 cloves garlic, minced

½ cup snow peas

¼ cup coarsely shredded carrots

2 medium boneless, skinless chicken breasts, cut into bite-size pieces

1 teaspoon toasted sesame seed oil

- Mist a wok or large skillet with the oil and heat on medium-high until the oil shimmers.

- Whisk together the cornstarch, soy sauce, and vegetable broth in a large bowl.

- Add the vegetables to the wok in order of cooking time: mushrooms, onion, broccoli florets, ginger and garlic, snow peas, and carrots. Cook each ingredient 1 to 2 minutes before adding the next.

- When the vegetables are tender, remove them from the wok, add a fresh mist of oil, and add the chicken.

- Sauté the chicken for 3 to 4 minutes, or until barely cooked. Take the wok off the heat and stir in the broth mixture. Heat on medium-high and stir 1 to 2 more minutes, or until the broth thickens. Stir in the sesame seed oil immediately before serving.

# Green Chili with Chicken

**F** Fatigue

**I** Insomnia

**SERVES 4**
**Prep time:** 10 minutes
**Total time:** 35 minutes

**SERVING SUGGESTION**
Serve as a complete meal.

**RESET PHASE**
**MODIFICATIONS**
**ADRENAL RESET**
**Meal:** Lunch, dinner
**Modification:** None

**METABOLISM RESET**
**Meal:** Dinner
**Modification:** None

**THYROID RESET**
**Meal:** Any
**Modification:** None

**GLUTEN-FREE OPTION**
No modification needed

**VEGAN OPTION**
Omit the chicken and use
2 (12-ounce) packages
of tempeh, cut into bite-
size pieces, and use
vegetable broth instead
of chicken broth.

The flavor of green chilis comes from roasted tomatillos. If you wish to omit the salsa verde, you can buy 1 pound of fresh tomatillos, cut them in half, and roast them on a baking sheet for 25 minutes at 350°F. Add extra salt and cumin to taste.

Misting oil

1 medium onion, diced

4 garlic cloves, minced

3 chicken breasts, diced

3 teaspoons ground cumin

3 cups chicken broth

2 (15-ounce) cans cannellini beans and liquid

1 cup salsa verde

Garnish: ⅓ cup chopped fresh cilantro leaves

■ Heat a large saucepan on medium-high for 30 seconds and add a fine mist of oil to the pan.

■ Add the onion and reduce the heat to medium. Sauté the onion for 2 to 3 minutes, or until clear. Add the garlic and sauté an additional minute.

■ Remove the onion and garlic from the pan and add in the chicken. Sauté for 3 to 5 minutes, stirring often, until the chicken is cooked.

■ Return the garlic and onion to the pan and add the cumin, broth, beans, and salsa verde. Bring to a low simmer and cook for 20 minutes. Remove from the heat.

■ Garnish with the cilantro and serve.

# Foil-Baked Chicken and Radishes

**F** Fatigue

**HF** Hot flashes

**SERVES 4**
**Prep time:** 25 minutes
**Total time:** 45 minutes

**SERVING SUGGESTION**
Serve as a complete meal.

**RESET PHASE
MODIFICATIONS**
**ADRENAL RESET**
**Meal:** Any
**Modification:** None

**METABOLISM RESET**
**Meal:** Dinner
**Modification:** Serve
with a carb and without
additional fat.

**THYROID RESET**
**Meal:** Any
**Modification:** None

**GLUTEN-FREE OPTION**
No modification needed

**VEGAN OPTION**
Use seasoned dried tofu
in place of chicken.

Radishes are one of the most underutilized of the cruciferous vegetables. When baked, they become sweeter and liven up the flavors of anything else they are baked with.

Misting oil

4 medium chicken breasts

Kosher salt and freshly ground black pepper to taste

6 cloves garlic, minced

1 tablespoon peeled and minced fresh ginger

¼ teaspoon cayenne pepper

1 pound sweet potatoes, peeled and cut into ¼-inch slices

1 bunch (8 to 12) radishes, trimmed and cut into quarters

1 medium sweet onion, coarsely chopped

Garnish: ⅓ cup chopped fresh cilantro leaves

- Preheat the oven to 450°F.

- Tear 4 sheets of aluminum foil, roughly 12 by 12 inches. Lightly mist each sheet with the oil and place a chicken breast on each sheet. Salt and pepper each side.

- Add the garlic, ginger, cayenne, sweet potatoes, radishes, and onions evenly to each sheet. Fold the sheets, crimping the edges together to close them, lay all 4 servings on a baking sheet, and place it in the oven. Bake for 20 to 25 minutes, or until chicken reaches 160°F on a meat thermometer.

- Remove the baking sheet from the oven and open the foil. Garnish each with the cilantro and serve.

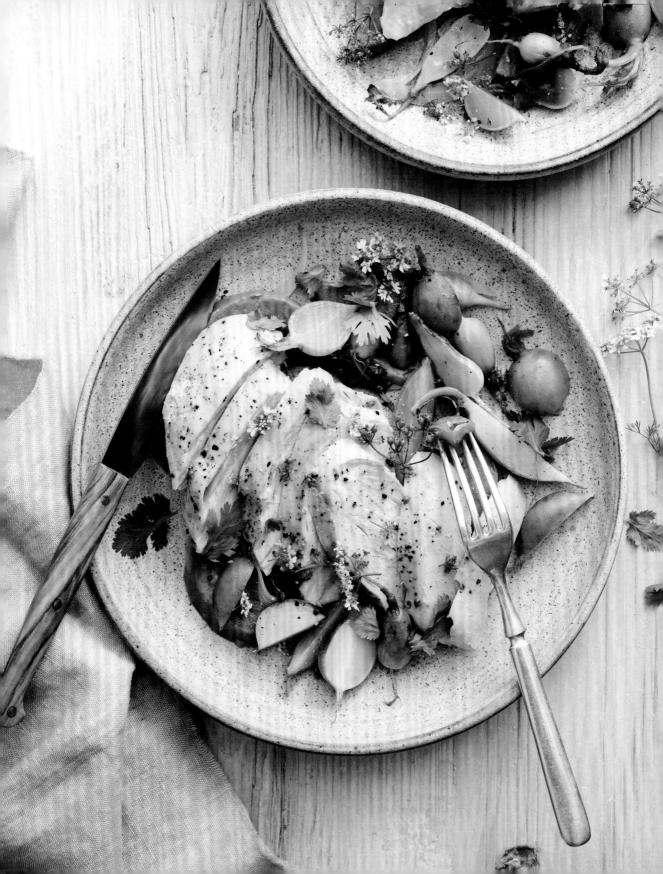

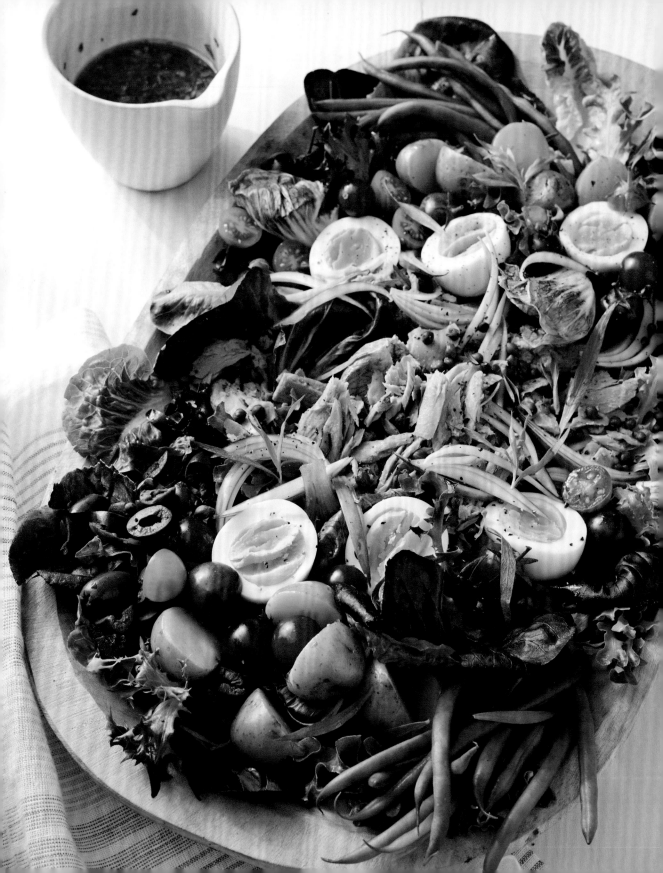

# Healthy Niçoise Salad

**SYMPTOMS IT CAN HELP**

**BF** Brain fog

**F** Fatigue

**HF** Hot flashes

**SERVES 4**
**Prep time:** 25 minutes
**Total time:** 30 minutes

**SERVING SUGGESTION**
Make this several hours
in advance, cover, and
refrigerate.

**RESET PHASE
MODIFICATIONS**
**ADRENAL RESET**
**Meal:** Any
**Modification:** None

**METABOLISM RESET**
**Meal:** Dinner
**Modification:** None

**THYROID RESET**
**Meal:** Any
**Modification:** Omit tuna
and include another
green-light source of
protein such as canned
chicken.

**GLUTEN-FREE OPTION**
No modification needed

**VEGAN OPTION**
Omit tuna and eggs.

This is an update on my prior Niçoise salad because I'm always trying to improve and simplify things. Rather than boiled potatoes, you can use leftover mashed potatoes and stir them into the dressing.

**SALAD**

2 (5-ounce) cans skipjack tuna, drained

9 hard-boiled eggs, peeled and quartered, yolks discarded if desired

1 pound Yukon Gold potatoes (2 to 3), quartered and boiled until just soft enough to pierce with a fork—usually 5 to 8 minutes

2 heads butter lettuce, washed, rinsed, and torn into small pieces

1 pint ripe cherry tomatoes, cut in half

1 red onion, thinly sliced

½ pound green beans, trimmed and cut into 2-inch pieces, blanched for 4 minutes with the potatoes

¼ cup kalamata olives

2 tablespoons capers, rinsed

**DRESSING**

⅓ cup lemon juice or red wine vinegar

2 teaspoons folic-acid-free nutritional yeast

¼ cup extra-virgin olive oil

3 tablespoons finely chopped shallot

2 teaspoons finely chopped fresh tarragon or 1 teaspoon dried tarragon

1 teaspoon Dijon mustard

Kosher salt and freshly ground black pepper to taste

- Combine the salad ingredients in a large serving bowl, with the lettuce as the base and the other ingredients in groups on top.

- Combine the dressing ingredients in a mixer bottle and drizzle over the salad just before serving.

# Lentil Veggie Soup

SYMPTOMS IT CAN HELP

F Fatigue

I Insomnia

W Weight gain

SERVES 4
**Prep time:** 10 minutes
**Total time:** 40 minutes

SERVING SUGGESTION
Serve as a complete meal.

RESET PHASE MODIFICATIONS
**ADRENAL RESET**
**Meal:** Any
**Modification:** None

**METABOLISM RESET**
**Meal:** Dinner
**Modification:** None

**THYROID RESET**
**Meal:** Any
**Modification:** None

GLUTEN-FREE OPTION
No modification needed

VEGAN OPTION
No modification needed

Lentils are amazing. They are so high in protein that they can provide enough protein and good carbs all by themselves. If you have some veggies, they can easily make a complete meal. They also cook faster than other legumes, are easy to digest, and taste great.

Other veggies can be added or substituted in this recipe—my wife likes zucchini in it. You can also take a little time and sauté the onions and garlic if you like.

2 tablespoons tomato paste

2 teaspoons kosher salt

4 cups vegetable broth

1 tablespoon lemon juice

½ medium onion, chopped

2 stalks celery, chopped

1 medium carrot, chopped

1 red bell pepper, seeded, cored, and chopped

2 cloves garlic, minced

8 ounces white button mushrooms, cleaned, stems removed, and chopped

1 (8-ounce) can diced tomatoes, drained

1 cup lentils, rinsed

1 bay leaf

1 cup chopped spinach leaves

Freshly ground black pepper to taste

- In a bowl, whisk the tomato paste, salt, vegetable broth, and lemon juice until well mixed.

- Pour the mixture into a large stockpot along with the onion, celery, carrot, bell pepper, garlic, mushrooms, diced tomatoes, lentils, bay leaf, spinach, and black pepper. Bring to a light boil over medium-high heat and simmer for 30 minutes, or until the lentils are tender. Remove the bay leaf before serving.

# Minestrone Meatloaf

SERVES 4
**Prep time:** 10 minutes
**Total time:** 70 minutes

SERVING SUGGESTION
Serve as a complete meal.
You can also refrigerate
for later use.

RESET PHASE
MODIFICATIONS
**ADRENAL RESET**
**Meal:** Any
**Modification:** None

**METABOLISM RESET**
**Meal:** Dinner
**Modification:** None

**THYROID RESET**
**Meal:** Any
**Modification:** None

GLUTEN-FREE OPTION
No modification needed

VEGAN OPTION
Use ground vegan meat.
Replace egg white with
liquid from the canned
beans.

Here is a fun take on a classic comfort dish that can help you get a good dose of garlic. All the expected minestrone flavors are in this dish, but in a baked form. I like to use 93% lean ground beef or plant-based ground "meat." For the oats, I typically keep old-fashioned in stock, but you can blend them dry in a blender for 30 seconds or so to get a texture more like quick-cooking oats.

Misting oil

1 medium yellow onion, diced

1 pound lean (93%) ground beef or turkey

1 (15.5-ounce) can cannellini beans, drained

1 (14.5-ounce) can diced tomatoes, drained

1 cup quick-cooking rolled oats

½ cup (precooked volume) small whole grain pasta like elbow or orecchiette, cooked and drained

1 cup diced vegetables such as zucchini, summer squash, or peas

1 tablespoon tomato paste

4 garlic cloves, minced

1 cup liquid egg whites

2 teaspoons dried oregano

1 teaspoon dried thyme

2 bay leaves

2 teaspoons lemon juice

1 teaspoon kosher salt

½ teaspoon freshly ground black pepper

- Preheat the oven to 400°F and mist a large sauté pan with the oil. Heat the pan on medium-high until a drop of water sizzles.

- Sauté the onion for 2 to 3 minutes, or until clear, and remove from the heat.

- Mix the onion with all the remaining ingredients in a large bowl.

- Mist a 9-inch loaf pan with more of the oil. Transfer the mixture into the loaf pan, spread it out evenly, cover with aluminum foil, and bake for 1 hour, until an internal temperature of 165°F is reached. Serve immediately.

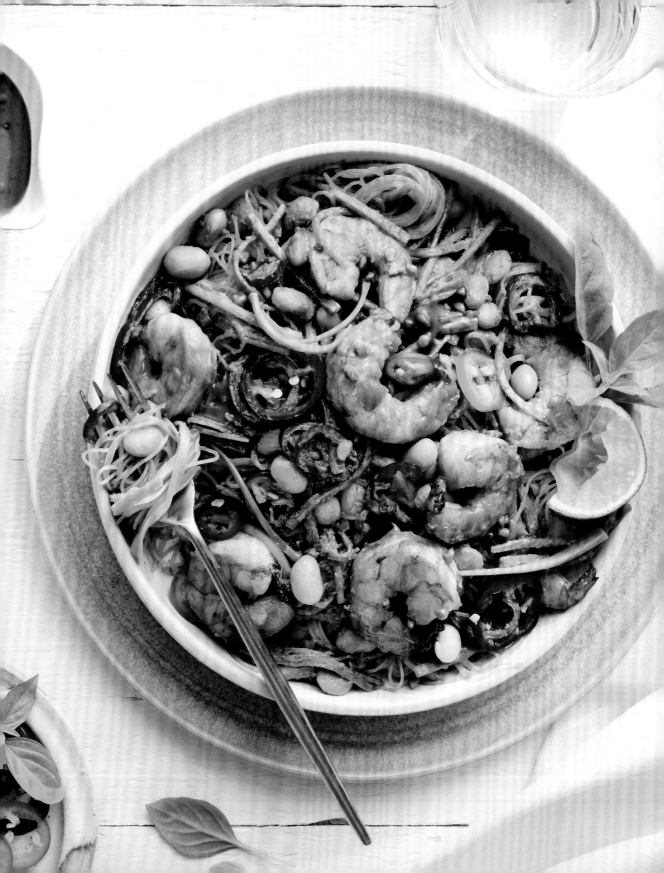

# Shrimp and Spicy Rice Noodles

SYMPTOMS IT CAN HELP

BF Brain fog

HF Hot flashes

W Weight gain

Shrimp is another good low-iodine version of seafood, especially when rinsed well. Adjust your use of the peppers based on your heat tolerance. If you like it hot, include the seeds and the membranes. If you don't like it hot, use only 1 or ½ of a jalapeño for the dish.

**SERVES 4**
**Prep time:** 10 minutes
**Total time:** 25 minutes

SERVING SUGGESTION
Serve as a complete meal.

RESET PHASE
MODIFICATIONS
**ADRENAL RESET**
**Meal:** Lunch, dinner
**Modification:** None

**METABOLISM RESET**
**Meal:** Dinner
**Modification:** None

**THYROID RESET**
**Meal:** Any
**Modification:** None

GLUTEN-FREE OPTION
No modification needed

VEGAN OPTION
Omit shrimp.

1 (12-ounce) package rice noodles

1 pound large shrimp, thawed, peeled, and deveined

Misting oil

2 cloves garlic, minced

1 large carrot, julienned into matchsticks about 1½ inches long

2 jalapeños, green or red, stems and seeds removed and chopped fine

1 cup frozen edamame, without pods

¼ cup crunchy peanut butter

2 tablespoons tamari soy sauce

1 tablespoon Sucanat or other natural sugar

Garnish: 1 lime, quartered

■ Soak the rice noodles in hot water per package directions. Soak the shrimp in the sink or a large pan with at least 1 gallon of water, swish shrimp around for 1 minute, change water, repeat, and drain.

■ Heat a wok or large skillet for about 30 seconds on medium-high. Lower the heat to medium and add a fine mist of oil. Add the garlic to the pan and sauté for about 1 minute.

■ Add the carrots and the jalapeños and sauté for an additional 2 minutes. Mix in the edamame, peanut butter, tamari, and Sucanat until blended and sauté for 2 minutes.

■ Raise the heat to medium-high. Add the shrimp and sauté until lightly pink and firm. Do not overcook. Add the drained noodles and stir until mixed evenly and the noodles are warmed. Serve garnished with the lime.

# Tofu Veggie Laksa

SYMPTOMS IT CAN HELP

BF  Brain fog

HF  Hot flashes

I  Insomnia

**SERVES 4**
**Prep time:** 10 minutes
**Total time:** 25 minutes

**SERVING SUGGESTION**
Serve as a complete meal.

**RESET PHASE
MODIFICATIONS**
**ADRENAL RESET**
**Meal:** Lunch, dinner
**Modification:** None

**METABOLISM RESET**
**Meal:** Dinner
**Modification:** None

**THYROID RESET**
**Meal:** Any
**Modification:** None

**GLUTEN-FREE OPTION**
No modification needed

This is a flavorful hearty vegan soup. The lemongrass is important. If you can't find fresh lemongrass, lemongrass paste is often available in produce departments. Dried lemongrass has almost no flavor and is not worth using.

2 tablespoons Thai red curry paste

1 teaspoon chili sauce

2 tablespoons tamari soy sauce

2 cups vegetable broth

1 cup canned light coconut milk

2 teaspoons folic-acid-free nutritional yeast

3 (4-inch) pieces fresh lemongrass or 1 tablespoon lemongrass paste

1 (8-ounce) package rice noodles

4 ounces white button mushrooms, stems removed, and quartered

1 zucchini, sliced

8 ounces firm tofu, cubed

8 ounces snow peas, ends trimmed

**GARNISH**

Juice of 1 lime

2 cups mung bean sprouts

- Whisk the curry paste, chili sauce, tamari, vegetable broth, coconut milk, and nutritional yeast in a large stockpot.

- Place over medium heat and bring to a simmer.

- Add the lemongrass, rice noodles, mushrooms, zucchini, tofu, and snow peas and cook until the noodles are tender, per the noodle packet instructions.

- Garnish with the lime juice and the mung bean sprouts and serve.

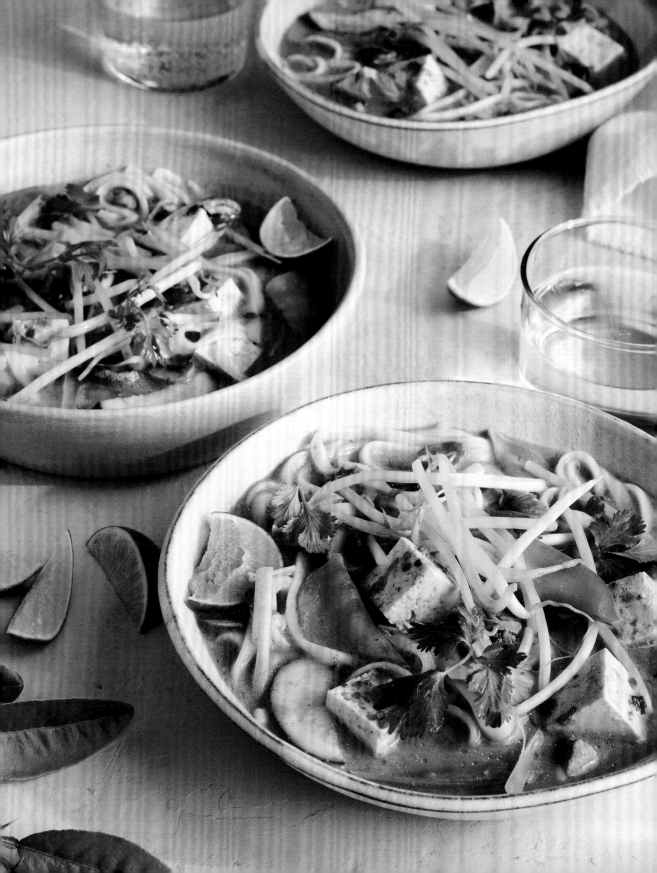

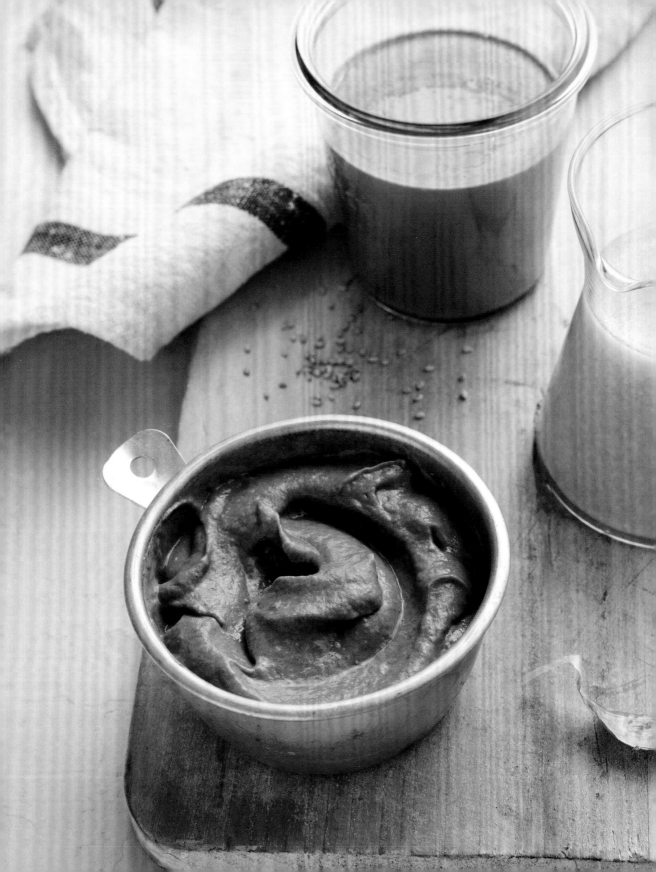

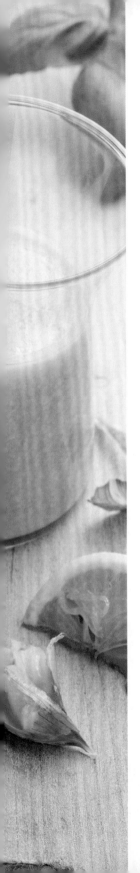

# Dressings & Sauces

You can use sauces along with most of the unseasoned protein and carb dishes. The dressings work well as options for variety on your Daily Salad (page 178).

**Avocado Spinach Pesto** 218

**Roasted Garlic Spread** 219

**Classic Walnut Pesto** 220

**Garlic Lemon Sauce** 222

**Sesame Soy Dressing** 223

SYMPTOM KEY

- BF Brain fog
- F Fatigue
- HF Hot flashes
- I Insomnia
- W Weight gain

# Avocado Spinach Pesto

BF Brain fog

F Fatigue

W Weight gain

**SERVES 4**
**Prep time:** 5 minutes
**Total time:** 5 minutes

SERVING SUGGESTION
Serve over pasta with cooked chicken and halved cherry tomatoes for a complete meal.

RESET PHASE MODIFICATIONS
**ADRENAL RESET**
**Meal:** Any
**Modification:** Serve in place of all other sources of fat.

**METABOLISM RESET**
**Meal:** Dinner
**Modification:** Serve in place of all other sources of fat.

**THYROID RESET**
**Meal:** Any
**Modification:** None

GLUTEN-FREE OPTION
No modification needed

VEGAN OPTION
No modification needed

If you have a hard time gaining weight, feel free to make this pesto with lots of oil and cheese in place of the avocado. I made this recipe because I love pesto but gain weight too easily. This pesto tastes as good as any classic recipes but with way more nutrients and fewer calories. If you are making it in advance, give the basil a quick blanch for 1 minute in boiling water followed by 2 minutes in a bath of ice water. This will prevent the color from degrading for as much as 3 days.

4 ounces fresh basil, stems removed, and patted dry

2 cups spinach leaves

1 medium avocado, peeled, pitted, and quartered

½ (15-ounce) can navy beans

½ cup aquafaba (liquid from the beans)

1 garlic clove, minced

Juice of 1 lemon

½ teaspoon kosher salt

¼ teaspoon cayenne pepper

■ Add all the ingredients to the bowl of a food processor or small blender, with the aquafaba and the avocado at the bottom. Blend until smooth and serve immediately.

# Roasted Garlic Spread

**BF** Brain fog

**F** Fatigue

**W** Weight gain

SERVES 8
**Prep time:** 5 minutes
**Total time:** 45 minutes

SERVING SUGGESTIONS
Serve as an
accompanying sauce to
any savory dish, especially
those with poultry or
tempeh.

RESET PHASE
MODIFICATIONS
**ADRENAL RESET**
**Meal:** Any
**Modification:** None

**METABOLISM RESET**
**Meal:** Unlimited food
**Modification:** None

**THYROID RESET**
**Meal:** Any
**Modification:** None

GLUTEN-FREE OPTION
No modification needed

VEGAN OPTION
No modification needed

Roasted garlic is nice to have in advance. Garlic bulbs are so small you can add them in the oven and let them cook anytime another savory dish is going. If you're turning the oven on for something else and you don't have any roasted garlic, you might as well throw some in!

4 whole garlic bulbs, unpeeled

- Preheat oven to 350°F.

- Slice the bottom ¼ inch off each bulb of garlic (the end with the root hairs), leaving the cloves intact.

- Place the garlic bulbs cut side up on a piece of aluminum foil. Wrap the foil around the individual bulbs and bake for 45 minutes, or until caramel in color.

- Let cool completely, then squeeze the roasted garlic out of the bulbs and into a small glass container. Serve immediately or store refrigerated for up to 1 week.

# Classic Walnut Pesto

SERVES 4
**Prep time:** 10 minutes
**Total time:** 10 minutes

SERVING SUGGESTION
Serve over whole grain pasta or zucchini noodles along with a neutral protein like diced chicken breast or sautéed crumbled tempeh.

RESET PHASE MODIFICATIONS
**ADRENAL RESET**
**Meal:** Any
**Modification:** Serve in place of all other sources of fat.

**METABOLISM RESET**
**Meal:** Dinner
**Modification:** Serve in place of all other sources of fat.

**THYROID RESET**
**Meal:** Any
**Modification:** None

GLUTEN-FREE OPTION
No modification needed

VEGAN OPTION
No modification needed

This version of pesto is lighter, with a cleaner and more concentrated flavor than most. Aquafaba, the liquid left over from cooking beans, is a perfect texturizer and source of resistant starch. The most typical way to get aquafaba is to open a can of chickpeas and pour off ½ cup liquid, saving the beans for later use. Choose walnut halves over chopped walnuts. The flavor is richer, since less of the oil is oxidized. In this version, the walnuts are well blended. You can also add them at the end and blend lightly if you'd like to preserve their texture. I love to serve pesto immediately after blending it. The colors and flavors start to fade immediately.

1 garlic clove, skin removed

⅓ cup shelled walnuts

Pinch of cayenne pepper

4 ounces fresh basil, rinsed, stems removed, and patted dry

½ cup aquafaba, with more as needed for food processor

1 tablespoon fresh lemon juice, plus more to taste

½ teaspoon kosher salt, plus more to taste

- Combine the garlic, walnuts, and cayenne in a small food processor or blender and blend until well mixed.

- Add in the basil, aquafaba, lemon juice, and salt. Blend until smooth and bright green. Add more salt and lemon juice to taste.

- Keep in the refrigerator for up to five days.

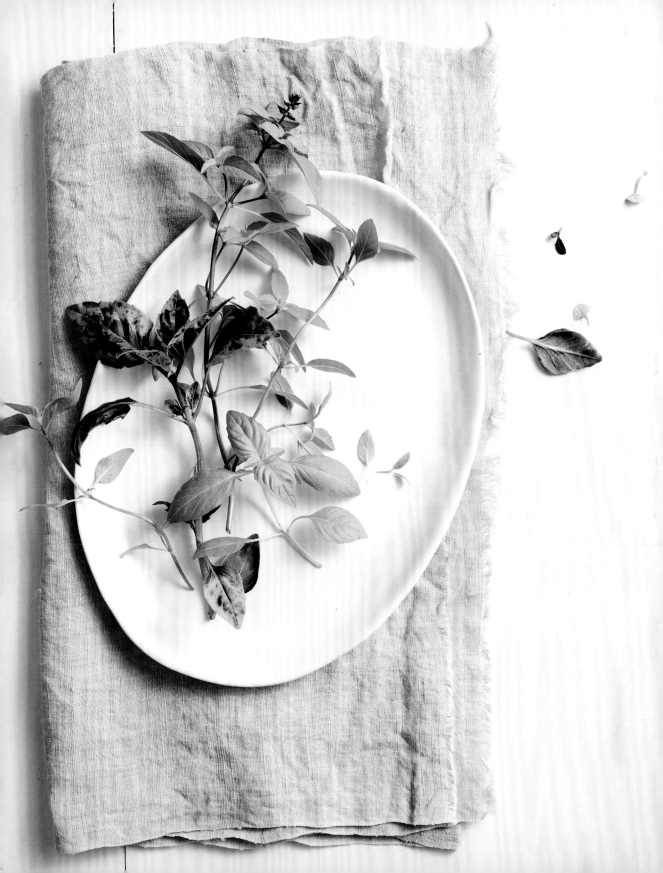

# Garlic Lemon Sauce

## SYMPTOMS IT CAN HELP

 Brain fog

F Fatigue

W Weight gain

## SERVES 4
**Prep time:** 10 minutes
**Total time:** 15 minutes

## SERVING SUGGESTION
Use as a fat-free salad dressing. Or top a spoonful onto your fish or chicken. You can also use it to top off your beans.

## RESET PHASE MODIFICATIONS
**ADRENAL RESET**
**Meal:** Any
**Modification:** None

**METABOLISM RESET**
**Meal:** Dinner
**Modification:** Serve in place of all other sources of fat.

**THYROID RESET**
**Meal:** Any
**Modification:** None

## GLUTEN-FREE OPTION
Use a gluten-free all-purpose flour like Bob's Red Mill.

## VEGAN OPTION
No modification needed

This is a modification of a traditional Lebanese dish called toum. It can be served with poultry, vegetables, or rice. This version uses much less oil and may need to be re-whisked after storage. Even though the sauce is blended, it helps to first mince the garlic. You can serve it right after blending, but it is even better if it is refrigerated for several hours or overnight!

⅓ cup minced garlic

Juice of 2 lemons
(4 to 6 tablespoons)

½ cup extra-virgin olive oil

1 teaspoon kosher salt

- Combine all the ingredients using a small bullet-style blender or food processor. Blend well for 2 minutes, or until an even consistency is reached.

- Serve immediately or refrigerate for up to five days.

# Sesame Soy Dressing

## SYMPTOMS IT CAN HELP

**F** Fatigue

**HF** Hot flashes

**W** Weight gain

## SERVES 4
**Prep time:** 5 minutes
**Total time:** 10 minutes

## SERVING SUGGESTION
Serve on a salad. Complementary ingredients include green leaf or romaine lettuce, diced avocado, mung bean sprouts, pea pods, cilantro, and bamboo shoots.

## RESET PHASE MODIFICATIONS
**ADRENAL RESET**
**Meal:** Lunch, dinner
**Modification:** None

**METABOLISM RESET**
**Meal:** Dinner
**Modification:** Serve with a carb and protein and without additional fat.

**THYROID RESET**
**Meal:** Any
**Modification:** None

## GLUTEN-FREE OPTION
No modification needed

## VEGAN OPTION
No modification needed

This is one of my favorite dressings of all time. It is easy to make quickly and can go on salads or noodle dishes. It can even be used as a stir-fry sauce. If you don't have a mortar and pestle, a food processor that can handle a small volume of food works as well. I like to make just enough to use, as the flavor fades when stored.

2 tablespoons raw sesame seeds

½ tablespoon Sucanat or natural sweetener of choice

2 tablespoons tamari soy sauce

2 tablespoons unseasoned rice vinegar

- Heat a medium-size skillet on medium.

- Sauté the sesame seeds, stirring frequently, for 3 to 5 minutes. When done, they will be golden tan and fragrant.

- Add the toasted sesame seeds and the Sucanat to a mortar and pestle. Grind thoroughly for about 5 minutes, until evenly mixed into a paste. Add the tamari and the rice vinegar and grind for a final minute until well mixed.

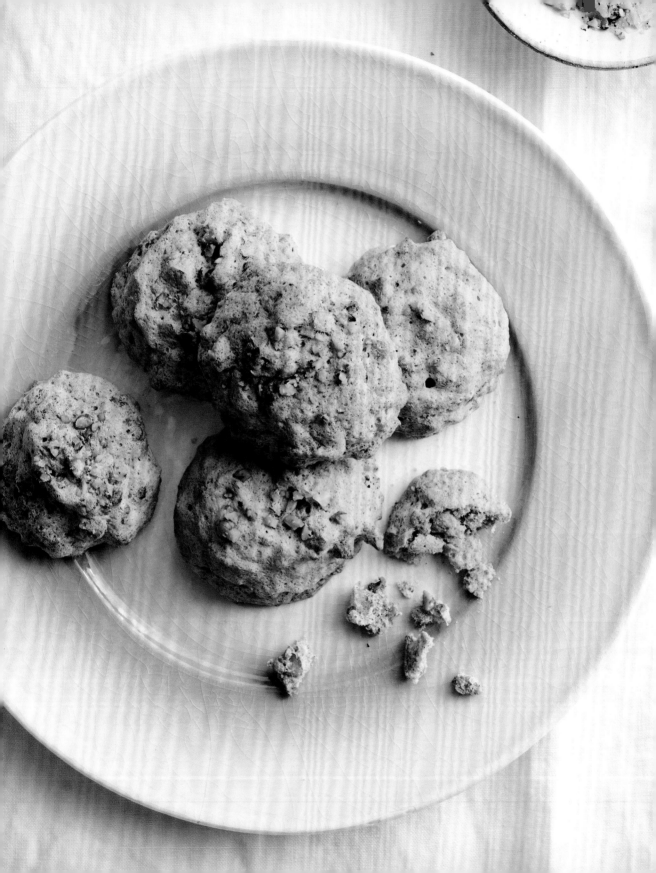

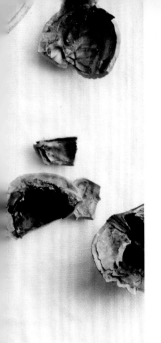

# Snacks

Here are a few odds and ends that use the same symptom-reducing ingredients.

**Walnut Cookies** 226

**Homemade Pickled Ginger**
227

**Toasted Pistachios with Chili**
228

**Rosemary Citrus Water**
230

SYMPTOM KEY

 Brain fog
 Fatigue
 Hot flashes
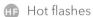 Insomnia
Weight gain

# Walnut Cookies

SYMPTOMS IT CAN HELP

**BF** Brain fog

**F** Fatigue

**MAKES 8 COOKIES**
**Prep time:** 30 minutes
**Total time:** 1 hour and 40 minutes

**SERVING SUGGESTION**
Serve as a dessert.

**RESET PHASE MODIFICATIONS**
**ADRENAL RESET**
**Meal:** Any
**Modification:** Serve in place of all other sources of carbs and fat.

**METABOLISM RESET**
**Meal:** Avoid
**Modification:** N/A

**THYROID RESET**
**Meal:** Any
**Modification:** None

**GLUTEN-FREE OPTION**
No modification needed

**VEGAN OPTION**
Omit the egg whites and add ¼ cup of flaxseed mixed into ¼ cup of water.

These are delicious, but bear in mind they are calorically dense!

2 egg whites

3 tablespoons Sucanat or natural sweetener of choice

1 teaspoon ground cinnamon

1½ cups chopped walnuts

- Preheat the oven to 350°F.

- Stir the egg whites, Sucanat, and cinnamon together in a medium bowl. Fold in the walnuts.

- Form into balls using 2 to 3 tablespoons of the batter and place on a baking sheet 1 inch apart.

- Bake for 10 minutes, or until lightly browned.

# Homemade Pickled Ginger

SYMPTOMS IT CAN HELP

**F** Fatigue

**W** Weight gain

SERVES 8
**Prep time:** 5 minutes
**Total time:** 45 minutes

RESET PHASE
MODIFICATIONS
**ADRENAL RESET**
**Meal:** Any
**Modification:** None

**METABOLISM RESET**
**Meal:** Any
**Modification:** None

**THYROID RESET**
**Meal:** Any
**Modification:** None

GLUTEN-FREE OPTION
No modification needed

VEGAN OPTION
No modification needed

Pickled ginger, known as gari in Japanese cuisine, is sliced ginger served with sushi. If you'd like to get more ginger in your diet, you can use this as a complement to nearly any meal. Just put a few slices on the side of the plate and experience the benefits of ginger every day! I like to make a double batch once or twice each month. As the mixture refrigerates, it often turns pink. This is a normal effect of rice vinegar on ginger.

½ pound fresh ginger, peeled

3 teaspoons kosher salt

1 cup rice vinegar

⅓ cup Sucanat or natural sweetener of choice

- Cut the ginger crosswise into thin slices. Place it in a bowl and stir in the salt to coat evenly. Transfer the mixture to a 16-ounce or larger heatproof jar and let sit for 30 minutes.

- In a small saucepan, stir together the vinegar and the Sucanat until dissolved. Bring to a boil, then pour the liquid over the ginger.

- Let cool, cover with a lid, and refrigerate for at least a week before serving. Store unused portions in the refrigerator for up to 3 weeks.

# Toasted Pistachios with Chili

BF Brain fog

I Insomnia

**SERVES 16**
**Prep time:** 5 minutes
**Total time:** 45 minutes

**RESET PHASE
MODIFICATIONS**
**ADRENAL RESET**
**Meal:** Any
**Modification:** None

**METABOLISM RESET**
**Meal:** Avoid
**Modification:** Best to
avoid nuts for snacks on
reset phase

**THYROID RESET**
**Meal:** Any
**Modification:** None

**GLUTEN-FREE OPTION**
No modification needed

**VEGAN OPTION**
No modification needed

These are good to have on hand to include as a garnish in other recipes or as an occasional snack!

1 tablespoon
fresh lime juice,
roughly ½ a lime

1 tablespoon
chili powder

2 teaspoons
garlic salt

1 teaspoon
ground cumin

2 cups shelled
pistachios, unsalted

- Preheat the oven to 350°F.

- In a medium bowl, whisk together the lime juice, chili powder, garlic salt, and cumin. Add the pistachios and stir until evenly coated.

- Spread the pistachios evenly on a baking tray and place on the center rack. Bake 25 to 30 minutes, or until the seasoning blend is dry and lightly toasted.

- Cool and serve. Keeps for up to 10 days in the refrigerator.

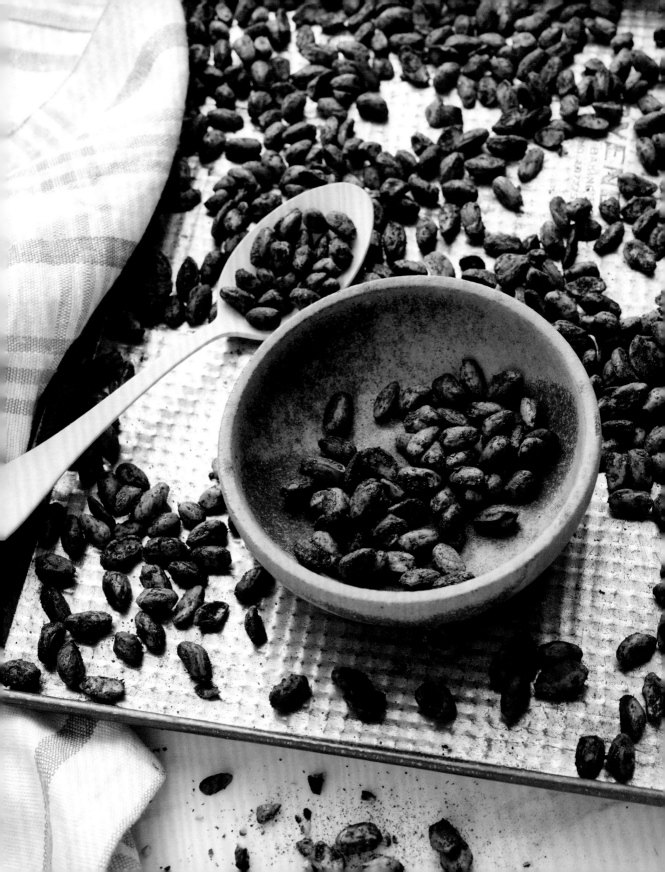

# Rosemary Citrus Water

SYMPTOMS IT CAN HELP

BF Brain fog

HF Hot flashes

I Insomnia

SERVES 4
Prep time: 5 minutes
Total time: 5 minutes

RESET PHASE
MODIFICATIONS
**ADRENAL RESET**
**Meal:** Any
**Modification:** None

**METABOLISM RESET**
**Meal:** Any–unlimited
food
**Modification:** None

**THYROID RESET**
**Meal:** Any
**Modification:** None

GLUTEN-FREE OPTION
No modification needed

VEGAN OPTION
No modification needed

This is the perfect beverage to help ease mental tasks. Much more effective than coffee, without the caffeine crash! I like to keep a pitcher of it on hand when I'm writing.

1 lime, sliced

1 orange, sliced

5 sprigs fresh rosemary

1 lemon, sliced

2 quarts purified water

- Add all the ingredients to a pitcher. Refrigerate overnight and serve.

# Endnotes

## Chapter 1: Hormones & Symptoms

1 Lorenzo Furlan, Christian Bonetto, Andrea Finotto, et al., "The Efficacy of Biofumigant Meals and Plants to Control Wireworm Populations." *Industrial Crops and Products* 31, no. 2 (2010): 245–54; doi: 10.1016/j.indcrop.2009.10.012.

2 Dagfinn Aune, Edward Giovannucci, Paolo Boffetta, et al., "Fruit and Vegetable Intake and the Risk of Cardiovascular Disease, Total Cancer and All-Cause Mortality—A Systematic Review and Dose-Response Meta-Analysis of Prospective Studies." *International Journal of Epidemiology* 46, no. 3 (2017): 1029–56; doi: 10.1093/ije/dyw319.

## Chapter 2: Food & Hormones

1 E. L. Lim, Kieren G. Hollingsworth, Benjamin S. Aribisala, et al., "Reversal of Type 2 Diabetes: Normalisation of Beta Cell Function in Association with Decreased Pancreas and Liver Triacylglycerol." *Diabetologia* 54, no. 10 (2011): 2506–14; doi: 10.1007/s00125-011-2204-7.

2 Soo-Jee Yoon, So-Rae Choi, Dol-Mi Kim, et al., "The Effect of Iodine Restriction on Thyroid Function in Patients with Hypothyroidism Due to Hashimoto's Thyroiditis." *Yonsei Medical Journal* 44, no. 2 (2003): 227–35; doi: 10.3349/ymj.2003.44.2.227.

3 Xavier Pi-Sunyer, "The Medical Risks of Obesity." *Postgraduate Medicine* 121, no. 6 (2009): 21–33; doi: 10.3810/pgm.2009.11.2074.

## Chapter 3: Weight

1 Sarah Steven, Kieren G. Hollingsworth, Peter K. Small, et al., "Weight Loss Decreases Excess Pancreatic Triacylglycerol Specifically in Type 2 Diabetes." *Diabetes Care* 39, no. 1 (2016): 158–65; doi: 10.2337/dc15-0750.

2 Nithida Narang, Wannee Jiraungkoorskul, and Parinda Jamrus, "Current Understanding of Antiobesity Property of Capsaicin." *Pharmacognosy Reviews* 11, no. 21 (2017): 23–26; doi: 10.4103/phrev.phrev_48_16.

3 Mariangela Rondanelli, Annalisa Opizzi, Simone Perna, et al., "Improvement in Insulin Resistance and Favourable Changes in Plasma Inflammatory Adipokines After Weight Loss Associated with Two Months' Consumption of a Combination of Bioactive Food Ingredients in Overweight Subjects." *Endocrine* 44, no. 2 (2013): 391–401; doi: 10.1007/s12020-012-9863-0.

4 John Springer, "60 Days of Nothing but Spuds Leaves Advocate 21 Lbs. Lighter." *Today,* December 2, 2010; https://www.today.com/health/60-days-nothing-spuds-leaves-advocate-21-lbs-lighter-2d80555614.

5 S. H. A. Holt, Jennie C. Brand-Miller, Peter Petocz, et al., "A Satiety Index of Common Foods." *European Journal of Clinical Nutrition* 49, no. 9 (1995): 675–90; PMID: 7498104.

6 Natalia Dos Santos Tramontin, Thais F. Luciano, Scherolin de Oliveira Marques, et al., "Ginger and Avocado as Nutraceuticals for Obesity and Its Comorbidities." *Phytotherapy Research* 34, no. 6 (2020): 1282–90; doi: 10.1002/ptr.6619.

7 Vahideh Ebrahimzadeh Attari, Alireza Ostadrahimi, Mohammad Asghari Jafarabadi, et al., "Changes of Serum Adipocytokines and Body Weight Following *Zingiber officinale* Supplementation in Obese Women: A RCT." *European Journal of Nutrition* 55, no. 6 (2016): 2129–36; doi: 10.1007/s00394-015-1027-6.

8 Vahideh Ebrahimzadeh Attari, Mohammad Asghari Jafarabadi, Maryam Zemestani, et al., "Effect of *Zingiber officinale* Supplementation on Obesity Management with Respect to the Uncoupling Protein 1-3826A>G and ß3-adrenergic Receptor Trp64Arg Polymorphism." *Phytotherapy Research* 29, no. 7 (2015): 1032–39; doi: 10.1002/ptr.5343.

9 Mie Nishimura, Takato Muro, Masuko Kobori, et al., "Effect of Daily Ingestion of Quercetin-Rich Onion Powder for 12 Weeks on Visceral Fat: A Randomised, Double-Blind, Placebo-Controlled, Parallel-Group Study." *Nutrients* 12, no. 1 (2019): 91; doi: 10.3390/nu12010091.

10 Gehan Elsawy, Osama Abdelrahman, and Amr Hamza, "Effect of Choline Supplementation on Rapid Weight Loss and Biochemical Variables Among Female Taekwondo and Judo Athletes." *Journal of Human Kinetics* 40 (2014): 77–82; doi: 10.2478/hukin-2014-0009.

11 Mahdieh Abbasalizad Farhangi, Parvin Dehghan, Siroos Tajmiri, et al., "The Effects of *Nigella sativa* on Thyroid Function, Serum Vascular Endothelial Growth Factor (VEGF)–1, Nesfatin-1 and Anthropometric Features in Patients with Hashimoto's Thyroiditis: A Randomized Controlled Trial." *BMC Complementary Medicine and Therapies* 16, no. 1 (2016): 471; doi: 10.1186/s12906-016-1432-2.

12 Ruth Nolan, Oliver M. Shannon, Natassia Robinson, et al., "It's No Has Bean: A Review of the Effects of White Kidney Bean Extract on Body Composition and Metabolic Health." *Nutrients* 12, no. 5 (2020): 1398; doi: 10.3390/nu12051398.

## Chapter 4: Fatigue

1 National Sleep Foundation, "Sleep in America Poll 2020: Americans Feel Sleepy 3 Days a Week with Impacts on Activities, Mood & Acuity." http://www.thensf.org/wp-content/uploads/2020/03/SIA-2020-Report.pdf.

2 Peter Maisel, Erika Baum, and Norbert Donner-Banzhoff, "Fatigue as the Chief Complaint—Epidemiology, Causes, Diagnosis, and Treatment." *Deutsches Ärzteblatt International* 118, no. 33–34 (2021): 566–76; doi: 10.3238/arztebl.m2021.0192.

3 Josef Finsterer and Sinda Zarrouk Mahjoub, "Fatigue in Healthy and Diseased Individuals." *American Journal of Hospice & Palliative Care* 31, no. 5 (2014): 562–75; doi: 10.1177/1049909113494748.

4 Neil Basu, Xingzi Yang, Robert N. Luben, et al., "Fatigue Is Associated with Excess Mortality in the General Population: Results from the EPIC-Norfolk Study." *BMC Medicine* 14, no. 1 (2016): 122; doi: 10.1186/s12916-016-0662-y.

5 Muqing Yi, Jinde Fu, Lili Zhou, et al., "The Effect of Almond Consumption on Elements of Endurance Exercise Performance in Trained Athletes." *Journal of the International Society of Sports Nutrition* 11 (2014): 18; doi: 10.1186/1550-2783-11-18.

6 Peng Song, Lei Wu, and Wenxian Guan, "Dietary Nitrates, Nitrites, and Nitrosamines Intake and the Risk of Gastric Cancer: A Meta-Analysis." *Nutrients* 7, no. 12 (2015): 9872–95; doi: 10.3390/nu7125505.

7 Norman G. Hord, Yaoping Tang, and Nathan S. Bryan, "Food Sources of Nitrates and Nitrites: The Physiologic Context for Potential Health Benefits." *American Journal of Clinical Nutrition* 90, no. 1 (2009): 1–10; doi: 10.3945/ajcn.2008.27131.

8 Meredith Petrie, W. Jack Rejeski, Swati Basu, et al., "Beet Root Juice: An Ergogenic Aid for Exercise and the Aging Brain." *Journals of Gerontology Series A: Biological Sciences and Medical Sciences* 72, no. 9 (2017): 1284–89; doi: 10.1093/gerona/glw219.

9 Joel Eggebeen, Daniel B. Kim-Shapiro, Mark Haykowsky, et al., "One Week of Daily Dosing with Beetroot Juice Improves Submaximal Endurance and Blood Pressure in Older Patients with Heart Failure and Preserved Ejection Fraction." *JACC: Heart Failure* 4, no. 6 (2016): 428–37; doi: 10.1016/j.jchf.2015.12.013.

10 Naoaki Morihara, Takeshi Nishihama, Mitsuyasu Ushijima, et al., "Garlic as an Anti-Fatigue Agent." *Molecular Nutrition & Food Research* 51, no. 11 (2007): 1329–34; doi: 10.1002/mnfr.200700062.

11 Seyedeh Parisa Moosavian, Zamzam Paknahad, Zahra Habibagahi, et al., "The Effects of Garlic (*Allium sativum*) Supplementation on Inflammatory Biomarkers, Fatigue, and Clinical Symptoms in Patients with Active Rheumatoid Arthritis: A Randomized, Double-Blind, Placebo-Controlled Trial." *Phytotherapy Research* 34, no. 11 (2020): 2953–62; doi: 10.1002/ptr.6723.

12 Naoaki Morihara, Mitsuyasu Ushijima, Naoki Kashimoto, et al., "Aged Garlic Extract Ameliorates Physical Fatigue." *Biological and Pharmaceutical Bulletin* 29, no. 5 (2006): 962–66; doi: 10.1248/bpb.29.962.

13 Anna Sjödin, Fredrik Hellström, EwaCarin Sehlstedt, et al., "Effects of a Ketogenic Diet on Muscle Fatigue in Healthy, Young, Normal-Weight Women: A Randomized Controlled Feeding Trial." *Nutrients* 12, no. 4 (2020): 955; doi: 10.3390/nu12040955.

14 Thomas M. S. Wolever, Maike Rahn, El Hadji Dioum, et al., "Effect of Oat ß-Glucan on Affective and Physical Feeling States in Healthy Adults: Evidence for Reduced Headache, Fatigue, Anxiety and Limb/Joint Pains." *Nutrients* 12, no. 5 (2021): 1534; doi: 10.3390/nu13051534.

15  Rajinder Singh, Subrata De, and Asma Belkheir, "*Avena sativa* (Oat), a Potential Neutraceutical and Therapeutic Agent: An Overview." *Critical Reviews in Food Science and Nutrition* 53, no. 2 (2013): 126–44; doi: 10.1080/10408398.2010.526725.

16  Rui Liu, Lan Wu, Qian Du, et al., "Small Molecule Oligopeptides Isolated from Walnut (*Juglans regia* L.) and Their Anti-Fatigue Effects in Mice." *Molecules* 24, no. 1 (2018): 45; doi: 10.3390/molecules24010045.

17  Luke J. Peppone, Julia E. Inglis, Karen M. Mustian, et al., "Multicenter Randomized Controlled Trial of Omega-3 Fatty Acids Versus Omega-6 Fatty Acids for the Control of Cancer-Related Fatigue Among Breast Cancer Survivors." *JNCI Cancer Spectrum* 3, no. 2 (2019): pkz005; doi: 10.1093/jncics/pkz005.

18  Steve Chen, Zhaoping Li, Robert Krochmal, et al., "Effect of Cs-4 (*Cordyceps sinensis*) on Exercise Performance in Healthy Older Subjects: A Double-Blind, Placebo-Controlled Trial." *Journal of Alternative and Complementary Medicine* 16, no. 5 (2010): 585–90; doi: 10.1089/acm.2009.0226.

19  Alain Jacquet, Adeline Grolleau, Jérémy Jove, et al., "Burnout: Evaluation of the Efficacy and Tolerability of TARGET 1 for Professional Fatigue Syndrome (Burnout)." *Journal of International Medical Research* 43, no. 1 (2015): 54–66; doi: 10.1177/0300060514558324.

20  Jordan M. Glenn, Michelle Gray, Lauren N. Wethington, et al., "Acute Citrulline Malate Supplementation Improves Upper- and Lower-Body Submaximal Weightlifting Exercise Performance in Resistance-Trained Females." *European Journal of Nutrition* 56, no. 2 (2017): 775–84; doi: 10.1007/s00394-015-1124-6.

## Chapter 5: Brain Fog

1  Suneetha Sampat, S. C. Mahapatra, M. M. Padhi, et al., "Holy Basil (*Ocimum sanctum* Linn.) Leaf Extract Enhances Specific Cognitive Parameters in Healthy Adult Volunteers: A Placebo-Controlled Study." *Indian Journal of Physiology and Pharmacology* 59, no. 1 (2015): 69–77; PMID: 2657187.

2  Negar Jamshidi and Marc M. Cohen, "The Clinical Efficacy and Safety of Tulsi in Humans: A Systematic Review of the Literature." *Evidence-Based Complementary and Alternative Medicine* 2017 (2017): 9217567; doi: 10.1155/2017/9217567.

3  Bo Kyung Lee, An Na Jung, and Yi-Sook Jung. "Linalool Ameliorates Memory Loss and Behavioral Impairment Induced by REM-Sleep Deprivation Through the Serotonergic Pathway." *Biomolecules and Therapeutics* (Seoul) 26, no. 4 (2018): 368–73; doi: 10.4062/biomolther.2018.081.

4  Adrian R. Whyte, Sajida Rahman, Lynne Bell, et al., "Improved Metabolic Function and Cognitive Performance in Middle-Aged Adults Following a Single Dose of Wild Blueberry." *European Journal of Nutrition* 60, no. 3 (2021): 1521–36; doi: 10.1007/s00394-020-02336-8.

5  Martha Clare Morris, Yamin Wang, Lisa L. Barnes, et al., "Nutrients and Bioactives in Green Leafy Vegetables and Cognitive Decline: Prospective Study." *Neurology* 90, no. 3 (2018): e214–22; doi: 10.1212/WNL.0000000000004815.

6  Mark Moss, Ellen Smith, Matthew Milner, et al., "Acute Ingestion of Rosemary Water: Evidence of Cognitive and Cerebrovascular Effects in Healthy Adults." *Journal of Psychopharmacology* 32, no. 12 (2018): 1319–29; doi: 10.1177/0269881118798339.

7  Yu Zhang, Jingnan Chen, Jieni Qiu, et al., "Intakes of Fish and Polyunsaturated Fatty Acids and Mild-to-Severe Cognitive Impairment Risks: A Dose-Response Meta-Analysis of 21 Cohort Studies." *American Journal of Clinical Nutrition* 103, no. 2 (2016): 330–40; doi: 10.3945/ajcn.115.124081.

8  Chung-Hsiang Liu, Chang-Hai Tsai, Tsai-Chung Li, et al., "Effects of the Traditional Chinese Herb *Astragalus membranaceus* in Patients with Poststroke Fatigue: A Double-Blind, Randomized, Controlled Preliminary Study." *Journal of Ethnopharmacology* 194 (2016): 954–62; doi: 10.1016/j.jep.2016.10. 058.

9  Jee Hyun An, Yoon Jung Kim, Kyeong Jin, et al., "L-Carnitine Supplementation for the Management of Fatigue in Patients with Hypothyroidism on Levothyroxine Treatment: A Randomized, Double-Blind, Placebo-Controlled Trial." *Endocrine Journal* 63, no. 10 (2016): 885–95; doi: 10.1507/endocrj.EJ16-0109.

10  Shinsuke Hidese, Shintaro Ogawa, Miho Ota, et al., "Effects of L-Theanine Administration on Stress-Related Symptoms and Cognitive Functions in Healthy Adults: A Randomized Controlled Trial." *Nutrients* 11, no. 10 (2019): 2362; doi: 10.3390/nu11102362.

## Chapter 6: Hot Flashes

1 Rebecca C. Thurston, Helen E. Aslanidou Vlachos, Carol A. Derby, et al., "Menopausal Vasomotor Symptoms and Risk of Incident Cardiovascular Disease Events in SWAN." *Journal of the American Heart Association* 10, no. 3 (2021): e017416; doi: 10.1161/JAHA.120.017416.

2 Anna-Clara Spetz, Mats G. Fredriksson, and Mats L. Hammar, "Hot Flushes in a Male Population Aged 55, 65, and 75 Years, Living in the Community of Linköping, Sweden." *Menopause* 10, no. 1 (2003): 81–87; doi: 10.1097/00042192-200310010-00013.

3 Francisco Fuentes, Ximena Paredes-Gonzalez, and Ah-Ng Tony Kong, "Dietary Glucosinolates Sulforaphane, Phenethyl Isothiocyanate, Indole-3-Carbinol/3,3′-Diindolylmethane: Anti-Oxidative Stress/Inflammation, Nrf2, Epigenetics/Epigenomics and In Vivo Cancer Chemopreventive Efficacy." *Current Pharmacology Reports* 1, no. 3 (2015): 179–96; doi: 10.1007/s40495-015-0017-y.

4 Xiaojiao Liu and Kezhen Lv, "Cruciferous Vegetables Intake Is Inversely Associated with Risk of Breast Cancer: A Meta-Analysis." *Breast* 22, no. 3 (2013): 309–13; doi: 10.1016/j.breast.2012.07.013.

5 Sarah J. O. Nomura, Yi-Ting Hwang, Scarlett Lin Gomez, et al., "Dietary Intake of Soy and Cruciferous Vegetables and Treatment-Related Symptoms in Chinese-American and Non-Hispanic White Breast Cancer Survivors." *Breast Cancer Research and Treatment* 168, no. 2 (2018): 467–79; doi: 10.1007/s10549-017-4578-9.

6 Ruwei Yang, Yang Zhou, Changbin Li, et al., "Association Between Pulse Wave Velocity and Hot Flashes/Sweats in Middle-Aged Women." *Scientific Reports* 7, article no. 13854 (2017); doi: 10.1038/s41598-017-13395-z.

7 Maryam Safabakhsh, Fereydoun Siassi, Fariba Koohdani, et al., "Higher Intakes of Fruits and Vegetables Are Related to Fewer Menopausal Symptoms: A Cross-Sectional Study." *Menopause* 27, no. 5 (2020): 593–604; doi: 10.1097/GME.0000000000001511.

8 Stéphane Zingue, Thomas Michel, Jules Tchatchou, et al., "Estrogenic Effects of *Ficus umbellata* Vahl. (Moraceae) Extracts and Their Ability to Alleviate Some Menopausal Symptoms Induced by Ovariectomy in Wistar Rats." *Journal of Ethnopharmacology* 179 (2016): 332–44; doi: 10.1016/j.jep.2016.01.004.

9 Ting-Ting Zhao, Feng Jin, Ji-Guang Li, et al., "Dietary Isoflavones or Isoflavone-Rich Food Intake and Breast Cancer Risk: A Meta-Analysis of Prospective Cohort Studies." *Clinical Nutrition* 38, no. 1 (2019): 136–45; doi: 10.1016/j.clnu.2017.12.006.

10 Xiao Ou Shu, Ying Zheng, Hui Cai, et al., "Soy Food Intake and Breast Cancer Survival." *JAMA* 302, no. 22 (2009): 2437–43; doi: 10.1001/jama.2009.1783.

11 Vilai Kuptniratsaikul, Piyapat Dajpratham, Wirat Taechaarpornkul, et al., "Efficacy and Safety of *Curcuma domestica* Extracts Compared with Ibuprofen in Patients with Knee Osteoarthritis: A Multicenter Study." *Clinical Interventions in Aging* 9 (2014): 451–58; doi: 10.2147/CIA.S58535.

12 Khatereh Ataei-Almanghadim, Azizeh Farshbaf-Khalili, Ali Reza Ostadrahimi, et al., "The Effect of Oral Capsule of Curcumin and Vitamin E on the Hot Flashes and Anxiety in Postmenopausal Women: A Triple Blind Randomised Controlled Trial." *Complementary Therapies in Medicine* 48 (2020): 102267; doi: 10.1016/j.ctim.2019.102267.

13 Kateřina Štulíková, Marcel Karabín, Jakub Nešpor, et al., "Therapeutic Perspectives of 8-Prenylnaringenin, a Potent Phytoestrogen from Hops." *Molecules* 23, no. 3 (2018): 660; doi: 10.3390/molecules23030660.

14 Naoko Ishiwata, Melissa K. Melby, Shoichi Mizuno, et al., "New Equol Supplement for Relieving Menopausal Symptoms: Randomized, Placebo-Controlled Trial of Japanese Women." *Menopause* 16, no. 1 (2009): 141–48; doi: 10.1097/gme.0b013e31818379fa.

## Chapter 7: Insomnia

1 Daniel J. Buysse, "Insomnia." *JAMA* 309, no. 7 (2013): 706–16; doi: 10.1001/jama.2013.193.

2 Ninad S. Chaudhary, Michael A. Grandner, Nicholas J. Jackson, et al., "Caffeine Consumption, Insomnia, and Sleep Duration: Results from a Nationally Representative Sample." *Nutrition* 32, no. 11–12 (2016): 1193–99; doi: 10.1016/j.nut.2016.04.005.

3 Ahmad Afaghi, Helen O'Connor, and Chin Moi Chow, "Acute Effects of the Very Low Carbohydrate Diet on Sleep Indices." *Nutritional Neuroscience* 11, no. 4 (2008): 146–54; doi: 10.1179/147683008X301540.

4 Rudolf M. F. Kwan, Susan Thomas, and M. Afzal Mir, "Effects of a Low Carbohydrate Isoenergetic Diet on Sleep Behavior and Pulmonary Functions in Healthy Female Adult Humans." *Journal of Nutrition* 116, no. 12 (1986): 2393–402; doi: 10.1093/jn/116.12.2393.

5 Ahmad Afaghi, Helen O'Connor, and Chin Moi Chow, "High-Glycemic-Index Carbohydrate Meals Shorten Sleep Onset." *American Journal of Clinical Nutrition* 85, no. 2 (2007): 426–30; doi: 10.1093/ajcn/85.2.426.

6 Indrakumar Sapna, Moirangthem Kamaljit, Ramakrishna Priya, et al., "Milling and Thermal Treatment Induced Changes on Phenolic Components and Antioxidant Activities of Pigmented Rice Flours." *Journal of Food Science and Technology* (Mysore) 56, no. 2 (2018): 273–80; doi: 10.1007/s13197-018-3487-1.

7 Justyna Godos, Raffaele Ferri, Sabrina Castellano, et al., "Specific Dietary (Poly)phenols Are Associated with Sleep Quality in a Cohort of Italian Adults." *Nutrients* 12, no. 5 (2020): 1226; doi: 10.3390/nu12051226.

8 Xiao Meng, Ya Li, Sha Li, et al., "Dietary Sources and Bioactivities of Melatonin." *Nutrients* 9, no. 4 (2017): 367; doi: 10.3390/nu9040367.

9 Glyn Howatson, Phillip G. Bell, Jamie Tallent, et al., "Effect of Tart Cherry Juice (*Prunus cerasus*) on Melatonin Levels and Enhanced Sleep Quality." *European Journal of Nutrition* 51, no. 8 (2012): 909–16; doi: 10.1007/s00394-011-0263-7.

10 Tai-Yin Wu, Wei-Chu Chie, Rong-Sen Yang, et al., "Risk Factors for Single and Recurrent Falls: A Prospective Study of Falls in Community Dwelling Seniors Without Cognitive Impairment." *Preventive Medicine* 57, no. 5 (2013): 511–17; doi: 10.1016/j.ypmed.2013.07.012.

11 Jack N. Losso, John W. Finley, Namrata Karki, et al., "Pilot Study of the Tart Cherry Juice for the Treatment of Insomnia and Investigation of Mechanisms." *American Journal of Therapeutics* 25, no. 2 (2018): e194–e201; doi: 10.1097/MJT.0000000000000584.

12 Hsiao-Han Lin, Pei-Shan Tsai, Su-Chen Fang, et al., "Effect of Kiwifruit Consumption on Sleep Quality in Adults with Sleep Problems." *Asia Pacific Journal of Clinical Nutrition* 20, no. 2 (2011): 169–74; PMID: 21669584.

13 Dawn M. Richard, Michael A. Dawes, Charles W. Mathias, et al., "L-Tryptophan: Basic Metabolic Functions, Behavioral Research and Therapeutic Indications." *International Journal of Tryptophan Research* 2 (2009): 45–60; doi: 10.4137/ijtr.s2129.

14 Mendel Friedman, "Analysis, Nutrition, and Health Benefits of Tryptophan." *International Journal of Tryptophan Research* 11 (2018): 1178646918802282; doi: 10.1177/1178646918802282.

15 FoodData Central Foundation Foods, https://fdc.nal.usda.gov/fdc-app.html#, accessed November 21, 2021.

16 Elham Oladi, Maryam Mohamadi, Tayebeh Shamspur, et al., "Spectrofluorimetric Determination of Melatonin in Kernels of Four Different *Pistacia* Varieties After Ultrasound-Assisted Solid-Liquid Extraction." *Spectrochimica Acta Part A: Molecular and Biomolecular Spectroscopy* 132 (2014): 326–29; doi: 10.1016/j.saa. 2014.05.010.

17 Darío Acuña-Castroviejo, Germaine Escames, Carmen Venegas, et al., "Extrapineal Melatonin: Sources, Regulation, and Potential Functions." *Cellular and Molecular Life Sciences* 71, no. 16 (2014): 2997–3025; doi: 10.1007/s00018-014-1579-2.

## Chapter 9: Recipes

1 Anna Maria Bertorelli and Roberta Laredo, "Serum Glucose and Insulin Responses to Sucanat and Sucrose in Non-Insulin Dependent Diabetes and Normal Controls." *Journal of the American Dietetic Association* 95, no. 9, suppl. (1995): A26; doi: 10.1016/S0002-8223(95)00442-4.

# Acknowledgments

I'd like to thank a few of the people in my life who made this cookbook possible.

Thanks to my lovely wife, Kirin Christianson. After twenty-six years, you're still my favorite food critic and kitchen helper. I hope to still be cooking with you until we are old and frail.

Thanks to my mom, Vivian Christianson. Mom often worked outside of the home, and our finances were usually tight. But I never wondered about dinner. We always had good homemade meals. Mom taught me that acts of service are the sincerest way to show love.

Thanks to my kids, Ryan and Celestina, for tireless feedback and patience with the many recipes that never got repeated. I love you both and I'm happy that you have kitchen skills and refined palates.

Alan Christianson
Hackensack, Minnesota
February 2022

# Index

# About the Author

Alan Christianson, NMD, author of the *New York Times* bestselling books *The Adrenal Reset Diet*, *The Metabolism Reset Diet*, and *The Thyroid Reset Diet*, is a naturopathic medical doctor who specializes in natural endocrinology with a focus on thyroid disorders. He founded Integrative Health, a physician group dedicated to helping people with thyroid disease and weight-loss resistance regain their health. He has been named a Top Doctor in *Phoenix* magazine and has appeared on national TV shows and in numerous print media. Dr. Christianson lives in Phoenix with his wife and their two children.

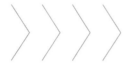

## ALSO BY ALAN CHRISTIANSON, NMD

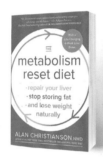

A four-week liver cleanse to help reset the metabolism.

A plan to help reverse the symptoms of thyroid disease by reducing excess dietary iodine.

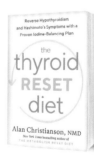

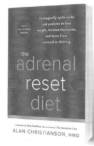

A plan to address three stages of adrenal impairment—Stressed, Wired and Tired, and Crashed—and get to Thriving.

**AVAILABLE WHEREVER BOOKS ARE SOLD**

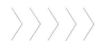

RODALE
NEW YORK

HARMONY
BOOKS